Dear World, Fibromyalgia people speak out.

Dear World, Fibromyalgia people speak out.

Everything you ever wanted to know about Fibromyalgia from the people who suffer from it.

Dawna L. Vance
with prayers by
Jan McDonald

Writers Club Press
San Jose New York Lincoln Shanghai

Writers Club Press
an imprint of iUniverse.com, Inc.

For information address:
iUniverse.com, Inc.
620 North 48th Street, Suite 201
Lincoln, NE 68504-3467
www.iuniverse.com

The names in the book have been changed to protect the inisent.
These are personal stories and I make no claims about medical knowledge.
It is intended for informational purposes only!

ISBN: 0-595-13427-0

Printed in the United States of America

Thanks to Jan McDonald for her prayers she wrote for this book.

Dedication

I dedicate this book to all the wonderful people who helped me to write this book with thier stories. I also dedicate it to my husband who has stood by me through the worst of pain and helped me to keep going.

Table of Contents

Dear World, Fibromyalgia people speak out.

Preface

I remember when I was going through the first signs of this disease. I went from doctor to doctor. If someone could of told me that there was a book or a place to go to that would of explained what was happing to me in terms I could understand, I would of jumped at the chance. You can ask your doctor a million questions but the best answers come from the people who suffer the same misary.

I spent a lot of time on the Internet in chat rooms and reading the message boards. What ever Internet service you are using, they should have a health section to look for a news groups or message board on Fibromyalgia. If you go to www.fibromyalgia.com or go to your search engine and type "fibromyalgia message boards". There will be a list of them there. You can learn a lot from the people who chat there. They are always ready to help anyone with any questions they can. I think because of the wonderful people I read about on the message boards was one of the main reasons I wrote this book. They are a wonderful group of people, who really care about each other.

Acknowledgments

I really want to thank all the wonderful people who suffer from fibromyalgia that sent me their stories. Because of your thoughts, ideas, and letters of encouragment we might bring some comfort to someone else.

Introduction

The stories you are about to read have truly touched my heart and I hope that they can somehow help you as well as touch your heart too. This is a collection of just a few people who deal with having FM every day of their life. If you thought that you were the only one who had symptoms or where the only one who felt the way you do the chances are there it someone here to relate too.

I have talked to people young and old and of all walks of life. With everyone comparing and sharing what is happening to them selves maybe it will help someone else who feels all alone. Believe me I too felt alone when I first started with symptoms and I didn't have anyone to go to or help me. I wish this book would have been around then, at least then I could have known I wasn't alone.

So I really hope this book helps someone who is feeling a little hopeless. We are out here and we do really care about what you are going through, because we too are going through the same things.

Chapter 1,

What is Fibromyalgia?

By now you probably know that FM is a widespread, chronic pain and fatigue disorder that has no known cure. Fibromyalgia means pain from mild to serve in the muscles, ligaments and tender tissues of the body. In addition to pain and fatigue, other symptoms include unrefreshed sleep, irritable bowel, chronic headaches, morning stiffness, cognitive or memory impairments, reduced coordination and decreased endurance. Although pain and fatigue are the two major symptoms, other symptoms may vary from person to person. Most popular complaints are: Muscular Pain: 100% Fatigue: 96% Insomnia: 86% Joint Pain: 72% Headaches: 60% Restless Legs: 56% Numbness and Tingling: 52% Impaired Memory: 46% Leg Cramps: 42% Impaired Concentration: 41% Nervousness: 32% Major Depression: 20%

The illness usually affects people between the ages of 20 to 60, often times striking when a person is in their 20's or 30's. It can however, affect people of all ages. Statistics show that 3 to 6 percent of the American population has symptoms that point to Fibromyalgia. It is estimated anywhere from six to twelve million people suffer from the devastating effects of this illness. Seventy five percent of suffers are woman. Even though there is not as many men they are out there and there are many children too. I read that the earliest detection in a child was 2 years old. How sad.

FM is usually something that happens all of a sudden so for most people is brings their way of life to a complete stop. The majority of FMS suffers are physically active, high achievers who live very productive lives. From the onset of the illness, the pain and fatigue impair a person from living the life they are accustom to. Many have to stop working, quit doing physical activities and even become socially isolated. The pain and fatigue can place a person in bed unable to function. Getting a diagnosis can be difficult. It usually takes 3 to 5 years to get diagnosed and then you have to spend thousands of dollars trying to figure it out. This disorder simulates many other things so it is hard for most doctors to diagnose it. Many patients are made to feel like "it's their fault", which undermines their self confidence and overall attitudes. People don't like being around a person who is chronically ill, so many lose the support of friends and family. Because of the lack of information about this disease most patients are unable to get any kind of disability. Supporting one's self becomes a major concern. Learning to live with irritating symptoms like constant pain, ringing in your ears, muscle spasms, concentration problems, and insomnia can be overwhelming. A sufferer of FM has to learn a completely new way of life.

If you have a history of widespread pain, and you wake up every morning feeling like you've been run over by a train, you may have FM. You may also have headaches or loss of balance can be a sign. Looking both ways when going into traffic can cause dizziness. Maybe you can't always find your car in a parking area. How about on your best days you feel like you have the flu. How about my favorite, you put on weight. Other signs are ridges on the fingernails, goose bumps behind the upper arms and thighs, and mottling of the skin. Sometimes you get muscle twitches. You might get a bad rash or hives. You might have allergies now when you have never had them before. You are electro-magnetically sensitive. Technically, you will have 11 of 18 specific "tender points". If these spots are pressed, you will have pain. However you could have pain today in 4 spots and 50 spots tomorrow. Fibromyalgia patients just about always have myofascial pain syndrome. You can't always depend on the 11 to 18 tender point system. These TPs are incredibly painful areas that often feel like knots or hard lumps in the muscles. Taut bands of fibers form in the muscles. The TPs refer pain to other areas. They can trigger gastritis, irritable bowel syndrome, grinding of teeth at night, pain when you put your hands in cold water, dizziness, weak knees, weak ankles, pelvic pain, dysmenorrhea and painful intercourse in women, vaginal dryness, impotence in men, and the list goes on. The tightened and spasming of the muscles can entrap nerves, blood vessels, and ducts. You can have blurring of the eyes or double vision. Leg cramps, hypoglycemic-like symptoms, problems swallowing, immune dysfunction, sensitivities, sciatica, numbness or tingling, mood swings, confusional states, loss of balance—the list goes on and on. So if this sounds familiar to you, then you just might be a fibromite!

Chapter 2,

An explanation of an invisable disability

Let me do a little explaining on how this diability effects a person on a day to day basis. As an outsider you may no what it is like to have sore muscles although I want you to know that your pain is not my pain. So don't give me some of your muscle relaxers because they won't work. I can't work through my pain and I can't shake it off. It's not even a pain that will stay put. It may jump from place to place. From shoulder to foot or arm to ankle. Some days I might not even have any pain at all. The reason that my pain is not like yours is caused by the mixed signals sent to my brain. So my brain can't tell if there really is pain or not. But I get the part of feeling terrible.

I get very clumsy at times too. If I wable when I walk or run into you, I don't mean to. I don't have good mucsle control anymore. My head spins round and round sometimes and I just can't stand still. So if you see me with bruises it is probably because I fell down not because I got hit.

I am useally so tired that that I am ofter near the state of servere exhaustion. I really might want to go do something with you but I just can't. But if you do see me out doing somthing phyical do think I am faking it. Because what I do today I will despratley pay for tomarrow. This is the price for stressing my muscles beyond their capablilty.

Then there is this thing we fibromites call "brain fog". It's not that I don't know who you are because we have been friends for 10 years, I just dont remember your name. My short term memory is so effected that sometimes if I don't write it down, then I can't remember even what I was going to say. I have posted notes all over the house just so I dont forget the important things in life like picking up the kids after school and where the school is. Ha ha.

I hate to say it but we all to often get moody too.This could be because we stress out on everything or everything stresses us out. Which makes the symptoms worsen. This often causes depression which again is just another mood swing. You get so tired of dealing with the symptoms that you almost get pushed over the edge.

I might be over wieght or I might not be able to gain weight but please dont point that out to me day after day. I can diet tell I am blue in the face but my appestat is broken and no body can tell me how to fix it.I dont choose to be this way and by loosing wieght it wont help the symtoms go away. My body gets so knotted up that exercising is about the last thing I can thing about. Infact the message that used to feel so great no is the most painful thing that I have to try and stand just to get myself functioning again.

Please don't tell me that your friend has FM and they are doing well or compare me with how bad they are doing. FM is different for everyone. No one is the same. We all have different gene pool make ups. So what one person feels or does is very different from another.

Now if by chance you see me on one of my good days, weeks or even months dont think I am cured. I suffer from a chronic pain and fatigue illness with no cure. But it is the days like these that give me hope.

I hope that this helps you understand this terrible disability. For the 10,000,000 people who suffer from Fibromyalgia they just want you to know how devastating this illness can be. Expecaily since they were once like you. Healthy and feeling fine one day and incapacitated the next with no worning. Please don't take these people lightly. You wouldn't want to spend even one hour in their shoes or their bodies.

Chapter 3,

Mind over Fibro

Dear World,

I have noticed that some people think it is a mind over matter, regarding the pain. I wish it were that simple. I am no shrinking violet. I have a very high tolerance for pain. Yet I am finding more and more days that I am down. I just don't sit at home thinking of my condition. I am out doing service for others and trying to be a good wife and mother. Just performing these simple tasks are enough to put me down lately. For the past 3 weeks I have been battling migraines and my stomach has also decided to cause me fits on top of all my usual pain. Still I keep trying to go but after a while, the body can take no more. I do get very offended when people say it is mind over matter. **It isn't !!!** I don't mean to bash anyone, but I just want to make it clear. If we find ourselves in bed for days, it's not our fault. We shouldn't be made to feel guilty. We have no control over the awful pain except to make it worse if we ignore the signs that tell us to slow down. We should be proud of what we can accomplish, and for the things we can't, oh well. I hope I don't offend anyone, but I just want to be understood.

Take Care,

L

Dear World,

You're so right, L—our mind can't do anything for FM—if it could, we certainly would **allow** "mind over matter!" I'm in your shoes, too—what a shame that **we** can't make social or civic commitments because we don't know how we're going to feel from day-to-day or, for that matter, from morning to evening and visa-versa! This is something "the others" don't think about! Last November I had to quit my beloved Women's Civic Club (leaving it without a very active vice-president. Boy, it hurt me so much to do that!) and not going around with my friends. A lot of them, but thank God not all of them, stopped calling because I always made an "excuse" that I couldn't go with them or do this or that. I miss all that very much. Fortunately, my **very best friend** is right here with me all the time, chauffeuring me around when necessary—I don't like to drive anymore; 10 miles wipes me out! So, yeah, you sure said a mouthful!!
J

Dear World,

It does seem like every once in awhile we get advised to "just put it out of your mind"," adopt a positive attitude" blah,blah,blah. Well-intentioned friends, uninformed medical persons, overzealous folks with a "this cured me so it will cure you" attitude constantly chip away at us. Is the glass half full or half empty? If life hands you lemons, make lemonade…Well I'm sure the rest of you can come up with lots of other cute sayings about adopting a positive attitude. Bottom line here folks, is that we are all human, with all the human frailties and warts. No one is any one thing 100% of the time, we just aren't made that ways. So along with the maintenance of a positive attitude it is very important to also love yourself and allow yourself to be human.

Every one responds to situations differently, and there is no one "right" way for everyone. Be true to yourself.

Hugs

D.

Dear World,

I went to the doctor today and I was explaining my aches and pains. He kept asking me questions and I answered them. This went on and on for about an hour. I really thought it was going somewhere. I thought soon he was going to tell me he had a magic pill that would make me feel better. Pretty soon he says "Well I think most of your problems are in your head." He then gave me a prescription for a anti-depressant. He also said he thought I was depressed. I thought my mouth was going to fall to the floor. I was lost for words. After that he just shoved me out the door and said "I will see you in 3 months". I couldn't believe my ears. I just wanted to scream at him that this was not all in my head. It was everywhere else that hurt. I wish I could break his arm and say "Oh that doesn't hurt". Well anyway, I just went home, cried and decided to get a second opinion. These are the kinds of problems faced by fibromyalgia people everyday.

KK.

Dear World,

Just wanted to let u know I see the neurologist tomorrow. It seems like it has taken forever to see him. My hubby is taking me tomorrow, so maybe I will be treated halfway descent. I am in **so** much pain today. I hurt from my head to my toes literally. I can't hold a book very long because it hurts too much. I have to take breaks when typing on the computer. What is making me more

nervous than anything is that I have had chest pains on and off today and am disoriented. The medicines I am taking are not hardly helping at all. I'm still having the headaches and the sleep deprivation. I am hoping that the doctor will order a sleep study for me. I am also praying that they will be able to tell me why I've had blackouts and memory loss. Deep down though I think all testing will come back normal. I don't know if I can handle that, because the doctors and others who don't understand the illness will think I'm a head case. I just know that what I am doing is not living. I am really looking forward to the day when someone will find a cure for this. Until then I'll just have to bite the bullet and cope with it. Thanks for listening.
T.

Dear World,

My story is a real sad one. I had to have surgery because of the drugs I took for the Fibromyalgia. I just got home from the hospital and I thought I would tell you how I feel. I have to say that right now, the post op pain has eased slightly but I'm still exhausted, not sleeping well because of the pain and in the middle of an Fibromyalgia flare up—I hate this. I have Irritable Bowel Syndrome so unfortunately I can't have Ibuprofen or Voltaren. I can't have any of the NSAID type drugs because of severe bowel bleeding I had after using Voltaren almost continuously for 3 years. I'd been complaining about the bowel bleeding for months to various doctors and they said it was just a normal part of IBS. Finally my doctor listened and took me off the Voltaren (which was helping to relieve inflammation in my back and knees) and told me I couldn't have any more anti-inflammatories until my bowel was examined and possibly never after that. The bowel bleeding, which had gotten so severe that I only had to sit on the pot and blood would pour out. This stopped within a week of coming off the Voltaren—and this is after months of asking doctors about the long term affect of taking the various medicines I was on and being (falsely) reassured that there would be no problems.

I talked with the surgeon a couple of days ago and he said I will probably need a six month course of strong hormonal treatment to hopefully get rid of the endometriosis and that may bring on symptoms of early menopause. It's either that or put up with the agony each month and the endometriosis will only get worse if its let untreated. The FM seems to mean it takes so much longer recovering from everything. Sorry to be so long winded but it seems one health problem complicates another and I'm fed up with them all.

P.

Dear World,

I'm in lots of pain-sick of it all and feeling quite weepy and down. I'm so weary and painful and exhausted at the moment that even my home work study is hard to do, but I'm sick on relying on government handouts and not having enough money. I want to be able to earn some money by working from home eventually. I don't know how much I'll be able to do. The FM really gets in the way of planning for the future. I just have to take one day at a time and be flexible with anything beyond that. I'm really hoping that they find a cure for this or at least an effective treatment because I'm only 23 and don't want to spend the rest of my life like this.

I found with FM the symptoms can sometimes be frightening especially when you know that some of the symptoms you have are the same as other life threatening illnesses. It makes it hard getting the balance between ruling out other possibilities without being such a frequent visitor to health professionals that they stop treating you seriously. I just couldn't remember whether I took my pain killers when I got up an hour ago. I had to check the packet (I cut the strips into daily totals) and found I must have taken them. I Don't feel any better though. So I guess that tells me once again I've been put on next to useless pills. I only just saw my doctor yesterday for stronger pain relief. She said this should work, but I'm still in a lot of pain and too exhausted to keep fighting for something stronger. oh well that's life for me at the moment.

Love

C.

Dear World,

I thought I would share something interesting that happened this weekend. My family and my brother and his wife took my Dad and Mom out for lunch Sunday for my mom's birthday. I had been having a lot of problems for the last few weeks, but figured that if I took it real easy, I could handle it (yeah, right). The meal went well but when I went to stand up, I could hardly move. The pain was really intense in my hips and legs and it was all I could do to stand. I had to lean heavily on my husband and walk really slow just to get out of the restaurant. My family usually tries to pretend nothing is wrong with me and they were shocked to see what was happening to me. Part of this is my fault though. I didn't realize how much I tried to shelter them from my condition. Most of the time I only go over and visit when I am having a good day. They really had not seen me in that kind of pain before. Boy, what a wake-up call for them. For the first time, I could see they finally believed what I had been talking about. I think my stubborn, independent streak prevented me from letting them see how bad I could get because I didn't want any pity. I don't know if this will help them be more sensitive to my needs in the future, but at least they know now that it is not all in my head.

I have been using MSM lately and it seems to be helping the pain. My husband changed jobs recently and we have no insurance until July. I ran out of my meds which is probably why the pain started getting so bad again. The MSM really does help though, when I remember to take them. Forgetfulness seems to rule my life these days. Please keep me in your prayers while I get through these next three weeks until our insurance kicks in. I have to change doctors again because of it and hope to find one who knows about FM and CFS.

God Bless you all

O.

Dear World,

I think that as "Fibromites" we just want the world to understand what we are going through. When someone says "I have Fibromyalgia," we want the other person to have a understanding that what we have is real and can be very devastating. If I said "I have cancer," how would you feel then. Do you understand what I am getting at? It's not the sympathy so much but maybe some empathy. We want to be recognized in the world, just like any other medical condition. We want the world to be more educated on our condition so that when some one you know has these terrible symptoms, the world will understand.

Author

Being upbeat and optamistic

It's hard to be upbeat. But you know what? It's easier if a person was born like that and it's their nature. I sure believe in that. With FM it's like being two different people in one body: one side of me says "I want to do this—I want to do that—I got to do this—I got to do that" and the other side of us says, Ooooo, Noooooo! We aren't going to and that's that!" Fortunately for me myself, and I was born with good nature. I also have very strong, upbeat attitude ("I'm okay, you're okay"), very outgoing, people-oriented disposition, a high threshold of pain. I **think** I'm lucky that, most of the time, I listen to the positive side of myself and have the ability to fight the other side of me. But I do understand this isn't the way it is with lots of people. I wish that upbeat people could somehow tell the downbeat people the secret—but I'm afraid that's just how it is : some are, some aren't. But no matter which we are, FM has no favorites. All of us different kind of people (which makes the world go round) are all in the boat...FM is FM, period...and to what degree—or symptoms each of has, or has not—we have this monster standing over us. The best we can do for each other is "stick together" and figure out a way to get medical science to **really** listen to us. (Maybe it's because I am "upbeat" is why I don't have all the symptoms I hear about—huh?) Right now, I'm well into a flare—two days now—and I **think** I'll be out of it tomorrow...
J.

Dear World,

You asked what I do to help myself each day-I believe that every obstacle life deals me should be met with as much sense of humor as I can muster. This condition-the pain, the disabling effect on otherwise productive lives-lends itself beautifully to self-pity. I believe this to be the most disabling effect of all. I try to focus my thoughts on what I am able to do, a search for answers, creativity in solutions, and support to others. I still consider my circumstances to be **temporary** even after so many years. I believe in progress with eyes open to the possibility of complete recovery. I am not a fighter by nature but more like what is said of the bumblebee-I don't have enough sense to know I can not fly and I hope I never do.

Best Wishes W.

Dear World.

I want to share with you this piece of advice. I have had Fibro for most of my life, which makes it seem a very long time as I am 29. Most of it has been in pain. I finally feel that after the last 15 years that I have come to learn this. Believe me it has taken a long time to see the light. You only have one life (as far as we know anyway) so look after you. This does not mean that you have to be selfish, but to take an interest in what you are about, the inner you. Only you will know about you. This is no great philosophy, and probably sounds a bit goofy, but it works. When reading a book, or information on Fibro, don't just follow every word, take from it what you feel fits in with you, and your well being. When doctors and physicians tell you that drugs or antibiotics are the best or only thing for you, then get several opinions, and make your choice to make a decision, not theirs. You're the one that will be affected, by any decision made, and not them. Make sure that you have plenty of support, either a friend that you can talk too, or relative, partner. Having someone to understand, or try to understand you makes a lot of difference. When working, don't feel that you are a let down, just

because you can't do the things you used to. Learn to delegate, and let the environment you are surrounded by work for you. Life, really is stressful enough, without taking on board other peoples' problems. So try to avoid these situations and confrontations. Remember, you will be the one to suffer the longest after the argument has passed (flare up galore). If you can remember one thing it is this. You are in charge of you. There will be some tough decisions to make in your life. You're in control of the Fibro, it is not in control of you!
big Fibro hug to all
R

Dear World,

When I feel depressed, I go into my studio and play music. I love to sing and for some reason when I do it, it's just like the depression doesn't matter anymore. Even if you don't like to sing, I would suggest putting on your favorite music you like to listen to. It can be so up lifting. Some of us hurt so much, we can't even move to the music and sometimes I feel that way too. So then I put on my favorite music and I lay down on the bed and mediate to it. Just enjoy how wonderful it makes me feel. Sometimes I lie there and think of what it would be like to be well. You know, like what I would do if I could. I think about the trip I would take or even something simple like the meal I would cook. Then I have to think about the things I have to be lucky about. I think about what I can do and what I have. Just the simplest dreams can make me happy. We have to try to be positive. We have to think and plan a head for ourselves. Take small steps to achieve what we need to get done. Just do something every day to make yourself happy. A good Bath is always nice. Soaking can make you feel so much better.

Anyway everyone has something that they like to do just for themselves. So if you think of that you will have, it gives you something to look forward to every day.
Author

Dear World,

These are my idea's on where Fibromyalgia comes from. This had given me hope and I would like to share it with you. It works for me and there might be someone out there that it will also work for. So here is my life saver information:

Guaifenesin is a safe medication that is in the same family as some medications for gout, such as Benemid. The doctor that 'discovered' this treatment has Fibro, he is in practice in California and he is a professor of endocrinology. I have been on Guaifenesin since Sept of 99. This is a miracle, but it takes time, patience and you need to read all you can about this so you will understand why it works. There is a Internet support group of over 1400 people and they are also getting well. It is believed that Fibro patients have a genetic defect in the area of the renal tubules of the kidney. All people take in phosphates from food, etc., but the FM patient has a defective gene. This causes the body to put the phosphates back into the blood stream instead of the bladder. That's where they would be excreted out of the body. The blood stream will not allow the body to put the phosphates in the blood stream, (phosphates also interfere in the production of ATP-the energy cycle) The body then begins to tuck the phosphates in muscles and tendons. This causes pain on examination when these lumps are felt. Eventually we have the deposits all over our body causing tenderness and pain. When the level of phosphates rises (as they are taken back into the body instead of being excreted out) we tend to have the cycles of the flu feeling. Then once the deposits are settled in the muscles & tendons and fascia, we are tender to the touch-that bruised feeling. Guaifenesin causes the reversal of this process. The phosphates are slowly pulled out of the body and excreted. It is not something that happens over night, and often you feel worse while this is happening. But then as you purge your body of the phosphates, you will begin to feel better.

Your doctor or chiropractor will also be able to feel your body clear. I understand this much better than I can explain it, so please just read all you can on the subject. Guaifenesin some-times can be bought over the counter in 200 mg doses. There are a lot of doctors using this treatment and Guaifenesin is not expensive (it has been around for a LONG time). Guaifenesin is safe, little if any side affects.

My son has CFS/Fibro and he is also on Guaifenesin. He went through a time of feeling really tired but he is getting energy back. He really has not had pain, but he is showing the same symptoms I was when I was his age.

Also, buy the book "What your doctor may not tell you about Fibromyalgia" by Paul StAmand MD& Claudia Marek, RN. This book explains all about the protocol. This medicine has been my miracle and my only regret is not getting on it sooner. Take care and don't feel too overwhelmed, it took me a long time to understand this, and have faith in it.
P.

Dear World,

To all of you out there contemplating Guaifenesin…I just have to tell you about this.

I started Guaifenesin in January when I had hit rock bottom, wanting to literally give up and die. Here it is 4 1/2 months later and I am feeling so much better.

A few weeks ago I was dreading these 2 car trips because I didn't know how I'd feel. I live in Ky., my sick mother lives in Pa. I had to drive to Cleveland (5 1/2 hours away) last Thursday, and drive back down here on Saturday (to take my mother to the Cleveland Clinic...she saw a pain specialist for treatment of chronic pain...Fibro????) Anyway 5 days later, this past Thursday I drove 8 hours to Pa. to see her, then today, Sunday I drove 9 hours back down here...bad torrential rains made the drive even longer and more nerve-wracking. but...here's the good news...my body doesn't feel like I even sat for an hour...let alone all those hours.!!!! I stopped every hour and a half or so and stretched for a few minutes, but I did that before Guaifenesin too.

Before I started on Guaifenesin, I would take a road trip like that and I would stop and stretch every hour. Then load up on pain pills and be in absolute agony the whole time even after I arrived. I have been home now for about 3 hours...I feel perfectly fine...a little tired, but that is all...nothing else. Without the Guaifenesin I couldn't have done this. It has definitely made a difference in so many things. I was dreading riding in the car because I know how high the price was before. Now, that I see this big improvement I will definitely be making more trips.

Also, next weekend I have to make a plane trip down to New Orleans for an overnight trip for a work related meeting on Monday. I feel like Guaifenesin is really being put to the test and is passing with flying colors.!! Please, if you have tried everything else and it hasn't worked, give Guaifenesin some consideration. It does work...I am proof !!

H.

Dear World,

I have something good to say about Guaifenesin too. I just realized that my nails are all about 1/4 inch long and look perfect! Plus I have nothing on them. DR StAmand does say something in the book about nails and hair getting better. I also realized that I have been going most days from morning to night and not feeling too bad. Sometimes I have a pain here or there, but nothing like before. I am tired sometimes, but I have had a house guest (Friend of my sons) here for 3 + weeks and she is Japanese, doesn't speak much English. She was married to one of my sons' friends who turned out to be a big mistake. She left him and came here. She was pregnant and I had to get her to a clinic. There was so much to do and just the stress of having someone in your home (when you didn't expect it). Trying to get her visa checked, updated, flight changed, and a very emotional young girl to deal with. Of course, my son did a lot of this for her. Certainly it was all worth it, is was only 3 weeks out of my entire life and it made the world difference to her. Tradition is strong in that county, and her life would have been very different going back to Japan; no husband, and a half white baby. Not to mention the "already inflicted" emotional scars. She goes home on Thursday and I feel pretty good. I sleep well most of the time and often I've slept longer than I wanted to, but I was still tired. I have almost forgotten what the morning stiffness feels like. So far, that boundless energy some talk of, I have not seen. Although, last year, before Guaifenesin I would have been in bed or the couch and trying to figure out how to get to the bathroom. She goes home on Thursday, and on Friday we take the motor home and we're off camping for 4 days. We moved into this house 4 years ago because we thought we needed a small house, the other one was too big to care for. Now, we are looking for a new house, and a bigger house. I don't even have to worry about a 2 story because the steps don't bother me that much. Last year we had few plans, I was just trying to figure out how to get through the day. Our big trip was once a month to the doctor to get my prescriptions. Now, we go camping, got a bigger RV, and we are looking for a bigger house (with RV parking)! None of this would have been possible without Guaifenesin. I will forever be grateful to this protocol.

Yes, I tried it before and didn't follow the directions. I took the maximum dose and I was needlessly miserable. I need the lower dose. I found cosmetics that are Sal free and I stick with them. **This** time I followed the directions exactly. I only wish I had done it right the first time. **But**, at least I have done it!
B.

Dear World,

Sometimes I wish I had 3 wish's al though one wish would almost get me the other 2. However, even though these wishes are obtainable for most, they are not for me. I don't have the strength to get there. My first wish would be to have my health. From there I could get wish number 2. Which would be to make lots of money. And if I had wish number1, I would get wish number 3. Which would be to be thin, with a great body. So for those people who have their health, they just don't know how lucky they are. They have the chance to do anything they want in there life and get there. Most of them just don't realize it. I do feel lucky to have what I have but the dreams are fun. Your imagination can take you anywhere.
S.

Chapter 4,

Fibromites tell their stories

Dear World,

 I am a 33 year old with a body that feels sometimes feel like that of an 80 year old. I have always been active and always took pride in having it altogether. I am a neat freak who likes things in order and done on a timely basis. Slowing down has been a problem for me. I have always been active in sports. I played volleyball and ran track in high school. I was always busy doing something. I am married with three children, ages: 14, 10 & 2. They are all boys going in different directions. Trying to keep up with them is a task in itself. The older two are involved in many different sports and my toddler—well you know how toddlers are. I work part-time as a secretary and during tax season I am a tax consultant. My husband also works a lot of hours and is unable to help much with the kids.

 I think my first symptoms started after the birth of my first child. I had minor headaches and some fatigue. A few months after delivery, I had one of my ovaries removed. With the pregnancy of my second child, I became anemic and toxic. I had high blood pressure that put me in the hospital. After I gave birth, the trauma was too much for my kidneys. I lost my right kidney. It seemed as if I really never bounced back from my pregnancies and with each year that passed I felt worse and worse. I was tired of being tired all the time. I dealt with pain every day especially early morning and late at night. I had headaches almost every day, chronic ones at least twice a week. My hormones were out of whack. I was irritable all the time and my quality of life was terrible. I just didn't enjoy life anymore. I was very depressed.

With the birth of my third child—a huge surprise, but a great blessing—I knew there had to be something wrong with me, but what? Was I just born with a lemon for a body? Even playing a simple game of golf became a task. As stiffness and soreness increased, so did my score!

I heard about fibromyalgia from my sister-in-law who is an RN. I was telling her about my headaches and she said my symptoms sounded like FMS. So I did some research. I was amazed. I finally had a reason for all my pain. First reaction was delight to know I was not crazy. Second reaction was disappointment. There was no known cure.

My family, I would like to think they understand, but I really don't think they do. My husband—although he acts supportive—really just doesn't get it. On my bad days, he just doesn't know why I feel bad. He gets frustrated because there aren't any visual symptoms. I'm not bleeding, vomiting, have the diarrhea or running a fever so I must not be sick. My mother often asks, "What's wrong with your legs?" My brother thinks I'm just lazy. Yes, lazy. You know how much that hurts? I have gotten to the point I just pretend I don't have FMS. They ask what's wrong, I just pretend I don't know.

My general physician diagnosed me with FMS. He sent me to a Neurologist who was leaning more towards CFS (Chronic Fatigue Syndrome). The more research I did the more I found out that there are no set systems for FMS. I also have systems for SS (Seasonal Syndrome) and IBS (Irritable Bowel Syndrome).

My main symptoms are headache, fatigue, 18 tender points, confusion and pain in my joints.

I really don't know how I contracted it. It could have been the years of sports, gymnastics, my pregnancies or maybe it's been in my genes all these years. I do know if I aggravated my disease in my knees by a fall I had playing softball. Since then there are days I have shooting pain in my knees. At times I have difficult walking and if anybody was to touch my knees, especially on my tender points, it would be extreme pain.

My Neurologist's treatment was Triavil, an anti-depressant. This drug made me feel better than I had felt in years. I never realized how bad I was feeling until I started taking this drug. Almost everything has its bad effects and although Triavil was working it was also making me Miss Blimpie, the dreaded weight gain. So I tried muscle relaxers. These drugs made me nervous and created sleeplessness and constipation. I did however find one that helped, not depleted, but helped my systems. Then I decided to take a different route of treatment, the natural way— natural herbs, vitamins and antioxidants. I have yet to find any side effects and the results, although not as good as Triavil, are improving as I search for my perfect formula.

I really can't say I'm in remission. I still have very bad days, but my quality of life has improved greatly. I have recently weaned myself off of the muscle relaxers and seem to be doing OK with it. I cope with life one day at a time, try to stay active and look at life as a gift rather than a burden we must endure. I must say just writing this has helped my frame of mind.

My advice to anyone who suffers from FMS. Stay active. Don't let FMS win. I think if I were the type of person who wasn't a go-getter I would be suffering more than I am now. I would have given up. Especially since I feel I am going through this alone. If your family understands, great! Lien on them only when you need them. Don't become dependent on them. Just keep going. Pain or no pain. I'll leave you with a verse from the Bible. I learned it in Bible school, many years ago. I will always remember it. I have often referred to it when feeling overwhelmed. Maybe it will help you too.

"This is the day the Lord has given, let us rejoice and be glad in it."

Gentle hugs,

J.

Dear World,

Mine started a long time ago and is progressing over time despite all I have tried. Diets, exercise and medications. I have now started a new case for full disability on the bases of Fibro, stopping me from gainful employment. I have been tested at (UCP). United Cerebral Palsy Facility and they found me certifiable disable of holding down a job. The duration of testing was 20 days 2 hours a day covering many different forms of employment duties on different days' none of which I could endure. Which they would have qualified me for part time work if I could. I have been seeing the same doctor since 1985 and he is a known and respected Nurog/MD therefore I have along history documented. I was only diagnosed a year ago, although my doctor watched me carefully before he would tell me. One day I went into his office in tears over the fact my husband could not take having a wife always in pain, even when it came to making love. I was at my end and he said to me "you are not going crazy". "It is not your imagination." "You have **Fibromyalgia**." I was still crying as I looked up. Feeling somewhat relieved and still frighten. I was without words as my doctor continued to explain what Fibro is and it's history. When he finished I was still distraught. He came to me to comfort me. He went on to say that if I access to the library or the Internet that I should research it further so that I could understand what is happening to me. I went straight home and got on the net. Fibro was easy to find. As I read the pages it was as if I was reading my on pain dairy. Once again I have tried A-Z to just make it through each day. Every day brings pain some less or more than others. Up until four years ago I refused to accept the term handy cap but as time goes on I am very challenged with normal activities that before I never thought about I just did effortless.

Sincerely, S.

Dear World,

I'm 51 years old and I have had Fibro for the last 5 or 6 years. Although I was not diagnosed with it until last may, I also have arthritis in both knees. Since Fibro invaded my life I have had my world turned up side down. I used to work as a cook in a nursing home, and a daycare center. First I started having severe pains in my leg after I pulled my back moving a table. Then it gradually got worse. It got so bad, I could no longer stand or walk very far. The pain was horrible. It was a burning severe pain that goes all over my body. I can not do things like I use too. I'm exhausted most of the time, but I push myself and then I wind up paying for it. Depression does set in if I sit and think about the way I was and the way I am now. Even though I have a wonderful loving husband and family that keeps me going, I do not know why there is not more research done on this. I get barmbarded with quick fix remedies. Even though generally life goes on...the only meds I take for this is hydrocodene. I'm pretty much a shut in but I do venture out at times. If I go to the

store for a little while you can bet I will pay for it dearly later in the day and night. So good luck to you, may there be light at the end of this tunnel.
Love J.

Dear World,

I don't mind telling you how they concluded that I had Fibro. I was hurt at work and was treated for 7 years for this injury. After 6 surgeries, I still had upper back, lower back and arm pain. I started having stress attacks, my blood pressure shot up and I was put on all kinds of prescription drugs. My doctor—not the workman comp doctors—tells me that he believes I had Fibromyalgia. There was nothing that they could do about the pain, but give me pain medication. It did not work! I have had ulcers, irritable bowel syndrome, high blood pressure, stress attacks and constant pain! I wasn't looking for a way to help the fibromyalgia. I had constant diarrhea. I starting taking a new natural immune support drink mix, called—Bio Choice Immune Support, within three days my bowl problems were gone. In fifteen days, the pain from fibromyalgia was gone. I now do **not** take any drugs. No blood pressure pill, no pain pills, no problems with my ulcers and no tranquilizers. It's like rainbows and sunshine again.

Please tell all the women out there, that drugs do not help. They make other medical problems. They all need to know about a natural food immune support drink mix called Bio Choice. Everyone man, woman and child on this earth need to keep their immune system purring along with Bio Choice. If you think I'm kidding, go to this web site and read the studies done. You do have to make your own mind up, but for me, it's

the only thing that works. I truly believe in it. See Studies on—
Bio Choice Immune Support on the Internet.
Good Luck
B.

Dear world,

I am 33 and have been in chronic pain for 7 years. It started
with back pain and after three years of continuous pain, I had
back surgery. I had a spine fusion in my lower back with 5 rods
and 6 screws in my back. Sometime during my recovery, my
pain spread to my thighs and neck/shoulders. It then went into
my calves and upper arms. Two years ago my mom developed
lung cancer and was given 6 months to live. During this difficult time, my pain got worse and I was diagnosed with Fibro.

I am not sure how I developed it, or exactly when my
chronic back problems developed in the Fibro. In 94, my dad
died suddenly of a heart attack. I didn't sleep through a night for
almost a year—which I understand can be a trigger. I also was is
a car accident, which I suffered neck problems. Then, as I stated
above I went through a lot of stress during my mom's illness.

My Fibro has dramatically changed my life. Previous
to my chronic pain, I was very active—aerobics, biking, stair
master, racquet ball, weight lifting etc. Now I am struggling to
take the extra 55 lbs off that I put on from depression and lack
of being able to exercise. I have to work full time and get very
little understanding from my CO-workers. I sit behind a
computer all day, and must get up frequently to stretch. I don't
feel my friends or family understand how much this has
changed my life. I am trying to finish my education, but a
simple things like carrying a book bag and sitting in class can be
difficult. Most of my relationships with men have been strained

because I am limited in what I can do. Most men my age are still very active, and have a hard time understanding why I can't do many things.

My doctors drive me **crazy**! Several told me it was in my head (in so many words). It took them 3 years to get a MRI on my back! My surgeon told me (prior to being diagnosed. with Fibro) than I was flip-flopping my symptoms and I didn't want to get better. My rhematoligist doctor is OK, but contradicts what the specialists say in seminars—calling them quacks. I now am learning what works for me by trial and error.

With all that depressing news I do have some good news—I am getting better! For the first time in 7 years, I have pain-free moments. I have reduced my pain level by making many changes in my life—1 by 1. I made sleep my first priority. I go to bed at the same time every night. I drink lots of water, liquid minerals, multi-vitamins and calcium chew daily. I changed my nutrition to a more balanced diet, eating protein at each meal and lots of fruits and veggies. I limit pop, caffeine and food chemicals. I take Elavil at night, and Ambien once in a while. On my worst days I also take Flexural and Vicoden (now only about twice a month). I learned ways to deal with the stress in my life because this seems to be one of my biggest pain triggers. I go to physical therapy every few months when my pain level goes up. At last, but not least, I had to learn to pace myself and accept that I can no longer push myself the way I use to. It has been difficult to maintain some of these things, but I have probably become 70% better—which is well worth the effort!

To the author, I am very glad to hear you are in remission, and hope to be on my way someday! Thank you for trying to reach the people who do not have computers. I did tried a few support groups prior to getting a computer, but found the ones

I attended too negative. I did learn however, that you can get better (something I never was told).
Take Care,
L.

Dear World,

I have been sick lately and very desperate. I have an appointment for the Fibro Study going on in Gainesville, Fl at the University. I think there are 6 studies in Fibro going on right now. A while back they did an experiment about hot plates performed by Dr. Staud. (if repeatedly placed on the hands of Fibro patients they felt severe pain where as the normal group did not have severe pain). Anyway, I go on the 6th for a 45 min interview. How close you live to Gainesville is a factor in whether you can be in their studies. The rheumy in charge is Dr. Roland Staud. I started taking Guaifenesin because I couldn't see being bed ridden for the rest of my kids' teen years. I did the research on the procedure and was on it for 3 days when the study people called. I came off the Guaifenesin that night because I want to be medicine free when I go for the interview. Just so you know I have Fibro symptoms real bad. By the second day of the Guaifenesin treatment I was in the most severe pain. The third day it was unbearable. According to the book that is exactly how the Guaifenesin is supposed to work. People can be in pain for months on this and then you are supposed to have good days interspersed with the bad days. Then the good days turn into weeks, weeks into months and so on. After I go for the interview I will see if it will be all right to go on the Guaifenesin and be in the study. If not, I will put the Guaifenesin on hold until I finish the study. I want to be in the study for all of our sakes. We need help! I will post my news if I have any on the Internet for all to see.

Hugs,

B.

Dear World,

Let me tell you a little about my current self first. I was born in 1972, in Duncan, British Columbia, Canada. I started getting fibromyalgia symptoms in March 1996 following an illness of Mycoplasma, a type of pneumonia. Even though the Mycoplasma was treated and went away, I was left feeling more and more troubled with my health. I do not believe I have Fibro…but one Doctor says I do, depending which one you talk to. One says it's all in my head and so does my husband.

My pain has been with me off and on for the past 10 years. At first the pain was in my back, it felt like labor pain. Nothing stopped it. I would run a fever at the emergency room too. They shook their heads, and said they could find nothing wrong. Once they wanted to do a spinal tap. (no way) I tried this bed, that bed, the floor, sitting up to sleep, even hanging half off the bed to sleep. **Nothing** works! I feel like I could do away with myself at times, because the pain is so bad, but I am a coward and could never do that. I even went to a shrink, who said I had no serious problems…So I have lived on drugs for who knows how long. I have worked, less and less, and my husband does not understand, and gives me little support. I decided to work more to be self supportive so I could leave him, what good is a man that does not have faith in you? He helped less and less…He even told my doctor recently that he thinks I get up tight and cause my own pain, in doing so. I have always been strong, rode horses, was a runner, worked out regular, did all the yard work, even when I was pregnant. Being a self employed person I would work around the clock.

I recall working 3 days and 2 nights straight. I assembled things, and sold them at art shows. I did 2-3 shows a week, stocking, mfg. the product, setting up for the shows, all long hard hours. The mfg. part is where I decided I got something toxic in my system that made me so sick, I still do not know. I refuse to give up my life although I do not work any more. I do this drug, that drug, and keep going. The pain is now in my back, neck, knees and legs. They all hurt at night, so I get very little sleep. In the past few months I have gotten what I call tennis elbow, and tennis shoulder, all on the left side. Can you believe it hurts to pull the cover up with my left side. How stupid, if it was not happening to me, I wouldn't believe the story myself. This is a person that's been a tom boy all her life, stacked hay, set up my own show booth, did walkways with 70Lb bricks, dug flag stone, etc. I have not bothered going to the doctor about this in a long while, he agrees with my husband. Flexural helps, and the doctor will not give me any more. He says I will get hooked. Huh? When I complain to the doctor (this is our primary doctor) he does not take me serious, so why bother.

I went to a bone specialist, they x-rayed me all over, bone scan, and they find nothing, SO, it's all in my mind. I have not bothered to go back. It **sucks**, and I am angry that I have trouble doing the things I love to do. I once ask for an arthritic drug and it swelled me up like a toad. That didn't help, so I quit it. I have been on Prozac for more years than I can recall. I stopped it about a month ago. I can go through a bottle of aspirin faster than anyone I know. My blood is so thin that I am cold all the time. One would think that with all the technology they have, they could fix me. Oh but as my husband says, "**mind over** matter." I do not mean to make him out to be a bad person because he isn't. He just has **never** been sick, had stitches or even broken bone…So what does he know.

Anyway, I do not know what else to do or say. I give up on vitamins and all that stuff that whoever says will help. I have tried lots of things, with little results. I cannot believe I have told you all this. I do not talk about it, not even my best friend does not knows of my pain. I have talked to no one about it. If I think or talk about it, I cry, if I don't, **maybe** it will go away. When I have a bad day, I don't answer the phone, take drugs or aspirin. I try to just sleep. I do know, I am getting weaker and weaker. So now I am going to try to take pain medication and work out to gain my strength. This is my new plan starting the first. I used to go 45min on the Nordic and do about the same with weights. I will not let this take away the things I enjoy the most, being active……Wish me luck.
R.

Dear World,

In 1985. I had all the symptoms…muscle pain, fatigue, headaches…actually thought I had lupus. Family doctor sent me to rheumatologist who diagnosed me with "Fibromyalgia." I would not die from this. Fine. I had 2 preschoolers, and went home and "forgot" about it…after all, there was nothing they could do, but give me and anti-inflammatory that upset my stomach. Thinking back, I did have a cytoscopy?…bladder "surgery," and a laperoscopy about that time. They put me to sleep both times…??

Nov. 1997, I had a hysterectomy for prolasped uterus (it literally fell out)!. The surgery and recovery was a piece of cake. So in January, when I thought I would be feeling "normal." I started this flu feeling, achy and tired. I wanted to sleep all day. I went back to work at my IRS seasonal job…8 hours on a computer. I had terrible pain in neck and shoulders, migraine headaches. I thought it was sitting at the computer, so I quit in April. The symptoms did not improve. I was diagnosed with fibromyalgia in May.

The doctor gave me Flexural (muscle relaxer) that made me really sleepy all day! He told me to do aerobic exercise 3 times a week!! I spent most of that summer in bed. In July, I had the brilliant idea to go to library to look this up. Brought home a dozen books!! I then tried the "herbal route," the "Guaifenesin route," the "no sugar, caffeine route" etc. etc. Nothing helped.

Aug. '98 , someone ran into the back of my car at a red light!! Whiplash!! Then I went to chiropractor. He helped some, except for extreme fatigue. I went to him for 8 months. The best thing he did for me was give me a **big** ice pack to put on my neck and shoulders!

I went back to IRS in Jan. 99, but realized I had arthritis in my hands, and could not type long periods of time…although I had cut my hours to 5 a day. I lasted until March, and then I took a leave of absence.

I spent the rest of the year just trying to keep it all together for my family, with **no extras** for me. There was no volunteer work, no teaching classes at church, no PTA…just tried to keep up with laundry and meals. I have 2 teenagers, and husband.

In Nov. '99, I met a woman with lupus. She told me about these "Thymic Formula" vitamins/+++ that she had been taking. She had been totally down for 2 years, but she looked like the picture of good health. She told me it would take 2 months to tell a difference. I almost gave up, at $39 a bottle…12 a day!! No difference at 2 1/4 months…but then…just as I needed it!!…something kicked in. I have been back at the IRS for 2 weeks. I am working 6:00 a.m. to noon. I have a new job that allows me to work on a computer for a while. I do a variety of things on it. The week before I went back, I told my friend that I did **not** know how I would drive there (25 min.), work, then drive back. I had already planned how I was going to get an alarm so I could sleep in my car during breaks!! Of course, I take a 2 hour nap when I get home! Then I still go to bed early and don't do much in between…this is more than I have been able to do in **ages**. I kept my pj's on all day Sunday (played hooky from church!!)!! It was rainy and I knew I needed "a day"!!!

That's my story. Hope it helps someone.

BJ

Dear World,

This is my story. I am a 49 year old female. I was officially diagnosed with fibromyalgia several years ago and immediately understood that I have suffered from it since I was six years old. It was almost a relief to get the diagnosis, in fact it was a huge blessing because I finally knew what really was wrong with me. It didn't stop the pain, but I finally knew what I had been battling. I won't waste your time by telling you all the avenues of recovery I have attempted. I'm sure they would be very similar to yours. When the rheumatologist had nothing to offer and an AMA internal specialist took me aside and said, "Medicine has nothing that can help you. Go and find alternative methods to ease your pain like, acupuncture, tai chi, or reflexology." I did all of that and more.

I went to an AMA allergist and immune specialist. I chose her because she has Fibro herself and was a brilliant researcher. She also believes in natural Vs chemical medicines. Under her care I was taking vitamin supplements (30, 3 times a day) and

Guaifenesin (1200 mg a day). After a year, I was definitely better but I still had a lot of pain.

One Saturday I was going out the door to refilled 10 or more bottles of supplements when a friend named Susan called. She said, "Please come over and meet my cousin Marla." She has Fibro like you and she found something that took away her pain." I was skeptical of course. I thought," well it can't hurt to hear her story." After all, we Fibro sufferers will try just about anything to get out of pain, right?

Marla had Fibro forever and the last five years she spent in bed taking every kind of pain medication imaginable. A friend brought her some Reliv Products. I looked at the can called Classic and said, "I tried this years ago. It doesn't work." Marla asked, "Did you take the Provantage, Innergize, Fiberestore, and Arthaffect with it at the same time?' I told her I hadn't heard of those products. Then she continued with her story. She said she drank three shakes a day (the product is in powder form). She said for three weeks she sat in a rocking chair and cried as her body detoxified itself from all of her pain medications. After three weeks, she felt energy returning for the first time in five years. After a month on the products she was pain free and fully functioning as a wife and mother of three for the first time in five years.

I bought the products instead of my supplements. That was on Sept 4th, 1999. I took them to my allergy/immune specialist and asked if she had ever heard of them.

She said no. I said "Good because if you had and they had worked, you would have told me about them." I then told her that I was going to commit to taking the Reliv Products for six months and stop taking everything she had prescribed completely.

She said, "Go ahead and try it, if it works, I'll buy some too" I mixed a scoop of each product with 10oz of distilled water and some ice, shook it up and drank it…three shakes a day. By the middle of October, I was pain free for the first time in my life. I did not experience the detoxification that Marla did because I had been taking supplements and no chemical drugs for a year.

I have since decreased the amounts of the scoops by half and only drink two shakes a day. I have incredible energy (I run a corporation). I sleep at night. I wake up without pain. I function as a normal healthy person. I go for long walks. I can do exercises with weights. In Nov 99 I fell down some stairs and severely sprained my ankle. I was in a cast and wheelchair for two months. The miraculous thing was I did not have a Fibro flare at all. Normally if someone so much as bumped into me, I would be thrown into a Fibro flare that could last for weeks. I had no soreness (except in the ankle, of course) even after a serious fall.

My daughter got a severe flu and was sick for weeks. Before Reliv, if someone so much as sneezed in the next room, I would get sick, the Fibro would flare and I would be in twice as much agony as usual.

I have spoken to people via the Internet and by phone who have taken these products. Every single one is a success story. Because these are patented, perfectly balanced food sources (not vitamin supplements) they produce amazing healing results for a large number of ailments.

I went back to my allergy/immune specialist after three months and she was amazed that I had no pain and no Fibro flares, fogs, etc., at all. (She got the product for herself.)

I personally know a chiropractor who has given up his twenty year practice to help people with Reliv because the products do so much more for people than he could do just being a doctor.

If you would like more specific information, go to www.reliv.com on the Internet. This product is sold through a distributorship.

I'm not sharing this to make money off of you. You can feel free to contact Reliv direct via the Internet. My main purpose in writing this is to send out a true, sincere message of hope. A lot of people have known my suffering and can't believe that I am no longer in pain, they are so happy for me.

There is so much more to this than I can write here. A forty year old woman who lived in the same town as I committed suicide because she could no longer live with the Fibro pain. That devastated me. That a life was ended because of this disease was so unnecessary. I will share with anyone who will listen the joy of being pain free. No one has to suffer from fibromyalgia.
Sincerely,
C.

Dear World,

Note to the Author—(Thanks for responding and I admire that you have the fortitude and strength to write this book.) We Fibromites fight and up hill battle for recognition and treatment.

How it started in my case, I don't really know. I had uterine cancer at the age of 38 in 1987. After the partial hysterectomy and chemo I became allergic to all substances very quickly even wool coats. I could wear a wool coat one month and I could not the next, carpeting, cats (although I had cats for 10 years) feathers, dust mites, molds, peanuts, almonds, etc. I was tired all the time. I even mentioned to a doctor that I thought I had Chronic Fatigue Syndrome. I was told there was no such thing. I still worked out regularly, tried to keep in shape. I had a career as a computer systems bank officer that was boring me stiff—but paid well. I was tired all the time susceptible to every germ—if someone sneezed; I got a cold, if a CO-worker had a cold I got bronchitis. My absenteeism was not good; I was still working 50 hours a week; seeing a chiropractor, allergist trying to treat my symptoms. I was also spending a fortune on vitamins, kyolic, etc. I was treated with Clarion, Emtex, Seldane, Naprosyn, etc.

In the spring of 1988 I was viciously attacked by a stranger when I was with friends. I had to have stitches on the back of my head and in my eye brow. My right eye was completely shut from the injury. I suffered whiplash and jerking. I mention this because some people feel that head and neck injuries are important in FMS.

Eventually, My career changed—I went to work in MIS at a non profit organization. I was recently married (1991—I married against all odds at 42). The reduction in stress I expected was not there; I worked 60 to 65 hour weeks but was paid well. I had surgery on my sinuses in August 1993 hoping that removal of polyps etc., would end my constant breathing problems. I developed asthma at 40.

After the surgery, I changed positions with a slight pay cut to another not for profit—it was supposed to be less stressful. I was fired after 6 mos. I simply could not keep up with the job. I took half of 1994 off and the first 6 months of 1995 to finish my Masters degree. I hoped to leave MIS and its crazy hours behind me and find administrative work. I was not able to so I became a part time adjunct professor in the fall of 1995.

Adjunct professors in New York work liked gypsies, moving from school to school teaching usually at 3 or more schools. Three part time jobs was the most I could handle I worked that way through 1996. In the fall of 1996 I began teaching at one school predominantly because the work was steady. I woke 28 hours a week with about 4 weeks off each year. I had suspected that I had lupus for years, having all the symptoms but kidney failure. During that time I saw the same physician for 5 years who gave me a vague connective tissue diagnosis and maintained on Prednisone. At first the shots were every 3 months; than every two months. Over the years I needed them more often. In August 1998 I heard about Fibromyalgia, read about it, and realized that was probably what I had. I contacted the national Fibromyalgia network and changed physicians. Not surprisingly the physician who previously treated me forwarded a very incomplete record not mentioning surgeries I had had or the Prednisone dosage.

In the early months of 1998 I was diagnosed with partial simple seizures and began treatment on Nuerontin; dosage increased from 300 ml a day to 1600 ml. a day. Body pain was increasing, insomnia was worse. I began to lose my previously excellent memory. I ran red lights when I drove because I did not notice them. I realized I could not work 28 hours a week and changed jobs to one where I worked 12 hours a week. The bending involved in teaching computer classes that were difficult. The stress phenomenal as I lost tests and assignments or never knew if students were lying or not. I finally realized this past December of 1999, that I could no longer work and am currently applying for disability.

I used to have an active social life, not any more. I am lucky that I have a wonderful husband who puts up with the fact that he must do most of the housework, cooking, and laundry. I am bedridden about 30 percent of the time and house bound about 70 percent of the time. I used to do walk-a-thongs for charity, including one that was 18.6 miles. Now I walk slowly with a cane and 6 blocks is painful.

Well that's my story and I hope it helps someone else feel not so alone.

Sincerely,

A

Dear World,

Let us begin-I had a normal birth 49 years ago. The only outstanding feature was the fact that my mother had RH negative blood and I am positive but no complications. As a child I suffered from allergies, bronchitis, swollen glands, and at 12 was diagnosed with asthma. There is no one-not even cousins-who have allergies on either side of my family tree. I was diagnosed with mumps at least 3 times-I think some may have been misdiagnosed. I fit into the category that has been discussed about polio vaccines-3 shots in 1955 later 3 oral vaccines given in the early 60's. We moved so often (Dad was military) I really can't attribute anything to environment.

As a child I was considered lazy. I made good grades but physically had little stamina. Although I rarely suffered asthma attacks and they were usually mild my lack of stamina was blamed on my asthma. I was pretty active, however ballet, swim team, bowling, I tried out for cheerleader twice but both times developed swollen ankles from jumping up and down. I went to college at 17 and began to have doubts of depression.

The first time I sought help for depression was after the birth of my daughter at the age of 23. I was given medication they no longer use because of fear of addiction-stellazine. It worked but I got off it very fast. In later years I worked, traveled, raised kids but I never could seem to keep up with my friends. A lot of the time when I tried I would come down with bronchitis. I think poor diet had a lot to do with it. Again I was called lazy.

At the age of 36 I gave birth to a son. Soon after I again sought help for depression. At this time I was diagnosed as manic-depressive or BI-polar and put on Lithium. I took it for about 5 years-the very min. dose, about 10 yrs ago. I began having severe pain in my stomach. At first, I was diagnosed with acid reflux. Over a year later with no relief I went back and it was discovered I had a hiatal hernia. Probably about a year later or less I remember thinking I was coming down with the flu. My muscles were tender and my skin was sensitive. It lasted only a few days and would come and go. I actually thought my immune system had improved and that I was successfully fighting off the flu because I never came down with it!

Another year later I decided to really get in shape. I was working out 3 hours. a day and looked pretty darned good however the muscle soreness I got from working out never went away even after 3 or 4 mos. Then I had a spell of dizziness at work but no cause was found. One of the pilots (I was a station manager for a commuter airline at the time) said he had had same problem and they had found a virus. Then we moved to Texas. I didn't work there and had severe bout of depression. Dr. said the lithium was being counter productive and puts me on Effexor. Effexor gave me bad headaches so I quit it after a few weeks and just toughed it out.

Then we moved again. This was about 5 years ago. I went to work mainly because of depression. I worked in retail clothing. I did lots of bending and stooping. After 4 months I began to get stiffer and stiffer as my shift wore on. I slept OK at night and the next morning no problems but again as the shift wore on I became stiffer and stiffer until one night I could not move at all. The muscles just would not respond. It was very frightening to me and the next day went to the doctor. Well, he did all the tests and only found I had hypoglycemia. He theorized that because of the hypoglycemia, lactic acid was building up in my muscles, I should make sure I eat on my breaks.

Then we moved again. I went back to work this time as a stocker and had no problems but only worked there 6 weeks. Then back to clothing sales. Another 4 months of bending and stooping and I was in so much pain I could no longer work. I quit and 3 months later went to a doctor who did more tests and said "I think you have fibromyalgia." He sent me home with ibuprofen-400mg, 3 times a day. By this time I had read a little on my own and I figured it was that or chronic fatigue syndrome. That was 4 years ago. The ibuprofen didn't do much except swell me up like a toad. I stayed home and took it easy.

Then last year in February I began to have some kind of weakness. I felt as I was going to faint but never did. I had missed a couple of periods and figured I was starting menopause, Dr. prescribed Prempro but after 6 weeks I was only getting worse and now was experiencing anxiety attacks. I went back to doctor and he prescribed Prozac. The first pill, 20mg-sent me into a major panic attack. Now I was getting to where food tasted awful and I was nauseated every time I ate. I hated taking baths or showers. Warm water seemed to smother me. Sleep was becoming increasingly difficult. I was becoming weaker and weaker and the tests showed nothing. The day before we left again, the doctor prescribed Xanax. The trip from Alabama to New Mexico is a blur. I was zonked out most of the time-nauseated the rest. Within a week of arriving here I was sent to Beaumont Army Hospital in El Paso-more tests. I had lost 20 lbs. in about 4 weeks and was beginning to realize I wasn't drinking anything either. They wanted to do an upper GI to look at my hiatal hernia and I just did not have the strength and began to pass out in the room. They rushed me into the emergency room but found nothing except I showed ketones in my urine so I was given IV dextrose. I could eat again! I got rid of all the pills and decided to get better on my own. I still had dr. Appointments however. Blood tests showed slight iron deficiency and I was given iron. Dr. in El Paso went over tests and said" Well, sometimes medicine just doesn't have all the answers." and left it at that. The doctor here in New Mexico is working with the doctor in El Paso and he said I was suffering clinical depression and had chronic fatigue syndrome. He offered no further help. He also said that my titer test for Lyme disease showed I had antibodies but no bacteria. This is still a mystery and I assume, at this point, the test was faulty.

By July I was able to drive again and very slowly getting better but continued to have flare ups. Sleep was still difficult. I had terrible headaches, possibly migraines, noise and light unbearable at times. I also had stiffness and soreness also extremely painful. I began to experience bowel problems, at times extremely loose and urgent need to go. My periods becoming less frequent. I had hair loss, Fingernails and toenails breaking easily. I had 5 teeth pulled because of gingivitis. I had blurred vision at times. Memory lapses and extreme fog.

Then at Christmas things seemed to be going pretty well. I had about 2 weeks were I felt OK. I was even thinking I might be able to go back to work. Then-Wham!!! I got a humdinger of a flare up. I was in so much pain! Just everywhere! I was disgusted with the Drs. at this point so I went to the computer and found the fibromyalgia board. I cried when I read all the stories of people like me. I was hoping someone had found an answer to the problem instead it broke my heart to read how many of us were suffering. After a couple of weeks of reading the posts I joined in. Somewhere during this time I read something about Sam-E. I always had a problem with the prescribed medication. I had been taking vitamins and supplements so I decided to try it. The first week I was on it I found I was becoming more optimistic but maybe that was because I no longer felt alone. In the next 2-4 weeks I realized my stiffness and soreness was beginning to subside. I was still having flare ups however. Headaches, soreness in my neck and shoulders from time to time. The pain seemed just below the surface as if it were waiting for me to make a wrong move. I was becoming more flexible but I was still having problems with sleep. I had been taking over the counter sleeping pills about 3 times a week but was worried about addiction when my daughter suggested Valerian. It worked beautifully-no hangover, no worry about addiction. I began to sleep well. My husband suggested I go hiking with him. He was very easy with me. We rested as often as I wished and came back home after an hour and a half. The next day there was no "pay back". I woke up one Saturday with terrible pain in my left shin. "Here we go again!" I thought. By 10:00 that night the pain was gone! A flare up that only lasted about 12 hours.? I could not believe it. My headaches were gone. My flare ups milder and shorter in duration. Maybe there was something to Sam-E.

Probably around the 6th week I was still having problems with fog-big time. I had tried Gingko Biloba before with no success but decided to give it another go. This time it worked. No more fog. By this time I am having no more headaches, very little stiffness, no pain. I am sleeping so well I do not need the Valerian anymore. I have one more hurdle-fatigue. I do not know if it's because I have been sedentary so long or if it's something else but I have yet to overcome the sometimes overwhelming fatigue.

Well, that's where I am at today. Still poking around the board and searching for answers. By the way, when I talked about pushing the cart-that was last year but my friend still pushes the cart for me now because as I said she still uses it as a walker. I can push my cart now with ease but I remember the pain and the stiffness. And because I am still afraid that one day I may experience another severe flare up I am cautious about saying I'm well. I'm not 100% and I don't want anyone to jump to the conclusion that I am. It is still early days. I have had steady progress but with this condition I know only too well that it could raise its ugly head at anytime and I might be back at square one. I knew this would happen if you got me started.

There is more. I have had a few injuries to my neck too. I mention this because of the latest findings about chiari? Malformations and the surgery they are now doing on some people. I suffered some physical abuse from my father, an ex-husband, and was involved in a rear end collision where I experienced whip lash but all were minor. I have never had major surgery. I didn't say all I should've about my flares or symptoms. After being diagnosed with Fibro about 4 yrs. ago and I had quit working-I found my left thumb would hurt from lifting clothes out of the washing machine. I thought I had sciatica because of pain in right buttock running down my leg. Sciatica runs in my family. I had pain in the top of my feet from time to time. Stiffness in my hips and knees sometimes caused me to limp or waddle. I have had pain in elbows, and my arms. A few weeks ago I developed a rash in the bra area. I have experienced pain in my chest causing me great concern about my heart and my left side seems to be giving me more problems now than my right. I have tingling in my arms and legs now if they are in a certain position-as if they are going to sleep and not getting enough circulation.

There is only one person in my family who has Fibro besides me. My cousin who is couple of years older who was burned severely over 65% of her body when she was about 8 or 9 yrs. old. This may account for her Fibro.

Well I think that is it. I hope it helps.

M.

Dear world,

Here is my story about Fibromyalgia. I felt to go a little more into my story for those who may have just been diagnosed or those who aren't even sure yet. It is a little lengthy but I remember how hard those first months were. I am hoping that this may help someone going through that process. I wish someone would have been there for me. Please feel free to share this with anyone who may benefit.

I first began having problems in November of 1991. It started with sciatic pain in my right leg and proceeded to get worse until it was all the way down to my foot. I was very stubborn and very involved in many things and refused to go to the doctor. By February of 1992 I had pain starting down my left leg to my knee as well. So I decided to go to a chiropractor who put me flat on my back, for several weeks and began very painful deep tissue work. By April my husband was getting concerned because I didn't seem to be getting better and he didn't have confidence in chiropractors to begin with.

That stated me on what I call my medical guinea pig journey. I was miss-diagnosed as having a ruptured disc. This was done without a MRI when I could pass all the normal tests. Since I had all these symptoms, you know that had to be the cause. So the answer was have an epidermal cortisone shot. I did not want to do this but, my husband and doctor were very determined that this would solve my problem. So the at end of

April I got the shot. Until that time I had only experienced pain in my hips and back of my legs.

The shot was pretty much painless and went very well, until the next day. I thought I was going to be paralyzed. The front of my thighs became hard as rocks and my pain got worse. I called the doctor panicked and he calmly said you just need to give it more time. Finally after continuing to get worse for 2 weeks he decided to order a MRI. Opps, I didn't have a ruptured disc after all. (I still had the bulging disc that I had had for years) but it wasn't any worse. So he decided that I needed to go for nerve impairment testing. $800 later the doctor gave me a prescription for physical therapy, an 8 page flyer on FM and told me I would learn to live with it. I had to come back every 3 week for a new prescription (another $80 visit).

I continued to suffer over the next 6 years. My trigger points in my upper body became activated (do to my new job). I survived on weekly sometimes BI-weekly deep tissue massage, getting in my hot tub daily, and a very supportive husband who had to take on a lot of extra work around the house.

Some days worse than others, depending on the weather, my level of activity, emotional stress, or whatever, day in and day out I was in pain from one degree to another. My emotions were also out of control, I was constantly sick, chronic sore throat, and bronchitis, any thing that went around I got, and I had it worse than most people did. By May of 1998, I was in so much constant pain, I was battling depression and had lost my desire to live. I was hoping someone would just put me out of my misery.

My nurse gave me a prescription for an antidepressant, which I took for about 3 weeks, but I struggled with taking a drug for depression. I was a Christian with a great husband, a good home why couldn't I just deal with it, why was I so depressed any way? Well, Chronic pain has a way of wearing you down day after day after day. When I went back the following month for my hormone shot she asked how I was doing on the drug. I told her I had stopped and why. What she did next has totally changed my life, I am so very grateful. She told me she had a friend who had also suffered and had experienced wonderful results with a new healthcare technology. She gave me her card, said I should talk to her, and that was it.

I called Amanda (her friend) and she told me the most remarkable testimony. I was very skeptical, but she told me this was either too good to be true or too good to pass up. She asked me if I was willing to risk passing it up and continue to go on the way I was, or was I ready to make a change? I now thank God I didn't pass it up or waste anymore precious time being skeptical. That was in June 1998, the following months have been the best I have ever had!!

At the time, I worked 3 days a week and that was all I could do. after work I collapsed on the couch in front of the TV, and my days off were spent there recuperating so I could work the next day. When I did do anything extra, I would seize up like the tin man left out in the rain. I started with intestinal support first for a week (I also had horrible bowel problems). Then I added the other Glyconutritional products. I kept a daily diary of how much I took and how I was feeling (which I highly recommend for everyone). It took me a couple of weeks to get a routine down and to find how much product I needed to take to get the results.

The first thing I noticed after a week or so, was a sense of well being, my desire to live returned, even while I still had the pain. The first correction my body started to make was my bowels. (I used to go 1-2 weeks without a bowel movement) That was normal to me and wasn't what I was looking for help with, but my body knew what was most important!!

Before my pain levels were constantly 7-12, now my bad days (which are very seldom) are 2-3 and I am walking 3-4 times per week in addition to a very busy and active schedule. If get a little sore I recover immediately, what would have taken weeks to overcome, I'm sailing through. I have a passion for life now.

I haven't had a hormone shot since January 99, and I'm doing great. I have gone 5 months without a massage. Now I'm on the go all the time, I share my testimony and these products every chance I get. Most of the time I get 6 hours of sleep or less by choice now, (but these are solid sleep hours—which I couldn't get before) I'm a true night owl by nature. I have so much energy, I feel so good and I'm continuing to get better and better.

I am so thankful for these wonderful products. They have changed my life physically, emotionally, spiritually and now they are beginning to change my life financially. (I now get my products free and am working full time getting this message to all who are suffering and looking to really change their life and take control of their own health. This has become such a mission for me that I have started a home business that I Call Daily Manna International. These nutrients are MY MANNA from heaven and everyone all over the world needs them especially if they have any auto-immune disorder like FM, CFS, Lupus, MS!

My heart is to help all those who are suffering without hope, and those who are looking for a natural alternative for optimal health and prevention. These nutraceuticals are my daily gift from God; HE has restored my soul, my health, and my hope. I turned 40 on 8/17/99 and it is going to be my best year.

I encourage anyone who's reading this and is considering these products, please don't hesitate, don't waste another precious moment suffering. Get started right away and commit yourself for 3-6 months, I promise you, you will be forever grateful. May your journey to health be blessed, it is an incredible trip!

Best of success to you,

SB.

Dear World,

I trace the start of my Fibro symptoms back to the pregnancy of my first son. I didn't really know what was wrong-I blamed all my symptoms on the pregnancy and working on my feet all day. It got worse with each successive pregnancy and never got better when I was no longer pregnant. So then I thought it was because I needed to lose weight. Well, after I lost 50 pounds and still hurt like hell. I went to the doctor. Five years later, I had my diagnosis of Fibro.

Good luck in your search for an answer.

N.

Dear World,

I gave birth to my daughter 6 months ago through C-section. I didn't really have any aches and pains throughout my pregnancy except for that last month. Then I had some swelling and stiffness when I move my fingers…something that lingered on 'till now. The worst part is that all of a sudden I woke up one morning and couldn't move my left knee. It felt so stiff and painful whenever I moved. I just took Tylenol and it would just ease up a little, but the stiffness and pain was still there.

This went on for 3 days. I was walking with a limp. A day after that painful left knee, I woke up the next morning with stiff neck and very painful right shoulder. I was not able to comb my hair. I had to keep my arm close to my body to control the pain,

I never felt pain like that in my life. Then the pain on my left knee went away but was only replaced with pain on my right knee. (You might not believe me but this really happened.) All the while with all the aches and pains, I had to take care of my then 6 weeks old baby who was still waking up every 4 hours for her bottle. Then as I suspected my left shoulder acted up, just the same way as the right. I was then breast feeding my daughter and I told myself that I couldn't take it anymore, it was just too much with all the pain and with taking care of her.

As sudden as they came, the pain on both shoulders and knees went away. Well, I still have the pain on my fingers and they act up once in a while, I have back pains now which I describe as burning pain. I hope to see a doctor soon and get answers for all of these.

Good luck to you!

Dear World,

I born in Glendale, California, on November 25th, 1969, raised the first few years of my life in silvery Hollywood, and transplanted to Midway City (AKA Little Saigon) around age 3.

I was a hyper kid, most of my friends were boys older than me and I played their vigorous boy games, "Cowboys & Indians," Cops & Robbers," Live Reenactments of Scenes From Star Wars with Fresh Fruit," etc. I loved sports and was very athletic. I excelled in softball, basketball, ran track & field, swam like a fish and received ribbons and trophies in all those fields. At the same time, I had allergies that were alarmingly difficult to reign in.

My folks schlepped me to GP's and allergists constantly. I had "scratch" tests that were like some form of archaic torture method. Still, I was fairly happy throughout. Heck, I was downright giddy! I had recurring sinus infections, scarlet fever, chicken pox…My mother was frantic in her attempts to better my health. She made my bedroom "sterile," removing carpeting and draperies and accouterments, & admonished me to not keep any thing aesthetic & not useful that would just "clutter" & "collect just."(Now I'm an artist/jewelry-maker specializing in creating things solely for their "aesthetic" value!)

The tide took a dramatic turn when I reached age 13. I slowed down, became fatigued, depressed, and withdrawn. Everyone just chalked it up to adolescence, but I believe now, that FMS was beginning to kick in. I remained lethargic & withdrawn throughout my teen years. I seemed to be feverish every day. I felt flu-like symptoms constantly. I withdrew into myself, into books & music. In my early twenties, I began to climb slowly, like a bear coming out of hibernation, out of my shell. Still without insurance or the financial resources to really delve into my condition, I soldiered on, throwing myself head-on into every activity I attempted. I always felt in the back of my mind, that something was really wrong, and that motivated me to make decisions and grab opportunities I wouldn't have otherwise chosen.

At a time when most of my friends were setting up house or pursuing degrees/careers, I took off across country by myself to explore for a couple months. I drove slowly up the whole of the West Coast, came to Seattle, and settled there for a while when I was 18. I've played guitar in bands & led the rock-n-roll lifestyle, partying until dawn. Then around my mid-20's, my condition began to change. I would be standing up straight, and suddenly, my knees would buckle and I'd fall. I'd go for a long walk, and find my legs in terrible pain the day after. I'd become disoriented easily. If a boss gave me a task, I'd forget the instructions within moments. I started to get scared. My parents speculated that it could be MS or Lupus, since they run in the family.

On a trip to Ireland in 1995, my health got so bad I couldn't walk for a couple days. I knew now that something was really wrong. Muscle pain and weakness increased. I became suicidal at times. I still was financially unable to seek a doctor's care. So I plowed forward. I got a full-time job in Torrance, and for the first time in my life, I got medical insurance. I saw a few doctor's until I got the diagnosis. "Fibromyalgia?" I'd never even heard of it! My rheumatologist' flip demeanor did nothing to allay my fears.

At the time of the diagnosis in 1997, there seemed to be a girth of information on FMS at libraries and bookstores. That has since changed. Back then, I was saved by Devin Starlynal's wonderful book on the subject. (Fibromyalgia and Chronic Myofascial Pain Syndrome.) I saw that FMS is a real disease and realized the extremity and complexity of the condition. I sought psychiatric counseling and my rheumatologist put me on Elavil. I felt no change in my condition after a few months on them. In fact, in a sense, I felt worse! I'd become a zombie! I tried Pamelor. Same thing I tried Flexural & Naproxen. No difference. Meanwhile, I was eating extra-strength Tylenol like candy to get me through the day.

I quit my job in 1998 and moved to London to be with my then-boyfriend/now-husband Chris, and there, my condition deteriorated. My symptoms ranged from blurred vision, to spasms, too intense all over muscle pain that literally brought me to my knees. After much deliberation, we left London for good, and returned to California, where the climate is milder.

I've managed to nurse myself back to a more livable state, with the aid of Chris & my parents. I'm taking care of myself holistically, using information I've culled from the Internet &

by trial & error on my person. I still need to get a lot of rest. I spend anywhere from 12-18 hours in bed daily, but I don't experience the devastating flares that turned me into a rampaging Neolithic huntress.

I have to use a cane occasionally, and I'm unable to hold a job. I've attempted to claim disability, and have been denied twice. I really don't expect to be able to secure disability, because these are the same people who denied my father disability last year, claiming his heart problems were not serious enough. He died of a heart attack on January 14th, 2000! It is my sincere hope to see FMS one day recognized by doctors and the media as the truly debilitating, curseful condition it is. Then and only then, will the suicide rate of FMSr's drop. We need our pain quelled and our voices heard.

Hope my story is of some use to someone somewhere.

Dear World,

I have 2 parts to my story. Hope they **help!**

S.

In 1988 my crippling symptoms of constant muscle pains, very low energy and horrific panic attacks began. I went from a high energy, healthy, working wife and mother, to a zombie like state! Doctor after Doctor told me it was all in my head. I knew I was slowly dying of some rare disease the Doctors could not find.

In 1991 I was diagnosed with Fibromyalgia, Chronic Fatigue and Panic Disorder. I was told they could only treat my list of growing symptoms because there were no cures. I was put on multiple medications for nine years, only to suffer terrible side effects that were personality altering and physically challenging.

My world became small and I was a stranger to my family! My hope of ever regaining my health disappeared.

In December of 1999 I was told it was in my head for the last time! I believe that I was misdiagnosed, over medicated, not listened to and labeled as unstable. Under the guidance of my Chiropractor I sought the advice of a Naturopathic Physician. My results have been incredible. When I began my journey just over 3 months ago now, I had a list of symptoms that was hand written on a full sheet of paper. Now my list has shrunk and my personality and hope for being healthy have returned! Small daily activities that normal people take for granted I now embrace. My husband and children never left me and for that I will be eternally grateful! My voyage is not yet finished, but if you can see yourself in my experience, and it gives you **hope** that's all that matters.

Here is the other part of my story.

I am very excited for you to get this information that helped me so much. I am over weight but have lost 20 pounds in the last 2 months doing just what the naturopath said to do! First I would like to start by telling you what meds I was on for 9 years. Xanax (anti-anxiety), Pepcid (for acid reflux), Doxepin (anti-depressant used in my case for sleep disorder for Fibro),Synthroid (hypothyrodism), Darvocet (every 4 hours for pain)Gaviscon (for heartburn)and Advil (for pain some-times used with the Darvocet or 600mg every 4 hours), and Zocor (a cholesterol lowering medication that did not work) I found out later I was not supposed to be on it due to my mus-cle disorder. People wondered why I was in such a Fog!

My breaking point came when I developed a metal taste in my mouth and could not figure out why for 2 weeks. I went to the MD and they told me it was nothing and to go home and relax. When I looked at my fee slip and he had written Panic disorder on it. I became outraged because I was not in a panic I was very calm and was just asking questions. By the time I got home I was in tears.

That night I found what was causing my metal taste. It was my earrings that I had left in the cleaner too long. I went to the Naturopath and found out that I have a main food intolerance, Which is dairy, and a second combination allergy that is fruit and sugar. I can have both just not within 6 hours of each other. I choose to have days when I have one or the other. It can get very complicated, but is so worth it.

I also found that I had a parasite in my blood. She said they are quite common in America today. I rarely checked for in the medical community because it is tropical and the only source that she can determine is the fruit that is shipped into our area. She prescribed an herbal remedy for that. My thyroid was not working hardly at all which did not make any sense to me because I had been on synthriod for 9 years. She said that because my body temp was always around 96.1 even in summer, and I had no reflexes below the waist and poor circulation the medication was not working. Your Body needs to be at least 98 degrees or your main organs have a hard time functioning. She also found that my adrenal glands were not working. I also was missing a very important tissue cell salt that is vital to life. I was also deficient in many other things, but did not find that until I requested a hair analysis.

I went for my first appointment. on Dec 30th 1999 and got my results on Dec 31st 1999. On Jan 4 2000 I started my new way of eating and the new thyroid(a natural hormone not synthetic) also the cell salts, seratonin and dopamine liquid, adrenal support and an herbal stomach remedy. It has been just over a full 2 month's time and I am off all of my Prescription meds except the Xanax. I needed to give my body a rest before moving on with that detox. I started to feel better almost immediately and have kept my clarity of my personality. no more fogs!

Now I'm not saying that I don't have bad days, they just don't put me in bed for days anymore. Based on how I feel now I don't think I had Fibromyalgia, Chronic Fatigue or the Panic Disorder. I recently had my cholesterol tested , after it being 405 in Dec. of 1999, it is now 228 21/2 months later.

All I did was get off of my many meds and changed my diet, excluding completely the foods that my body could not process. I go to a chiropractor 3 x a week which has also helped a lot. I can move and I have energy now. I know now that I am not nuts, and that to me is priceless! I was so bad that at one point a friend drove me to the hospital and admitted me to the physic ward for 2 weeks.

I have been through a lot in the last 10 years and now I'm on a mission to let as many people as I can know about my experience so they know there is another way and there is hope! Now I do not suggest that you stop taking any RX meds without supervision or that you start taking any herbs without supervision. Every **body** is different and needs individual care and attention and most of all **tender loving care.** You have to take the first step by asking for information. I hope you can find the determination to help yourself, because as I have painfully learned the hard way, no one will do it for you and there **are no magic pills.**

I wish you the best of luck on your journey!
"believe in yourself!" T.

Dear World,

I am 33, married with 2 beautiful children. I started having Fibro symptoms 2 years ago after my partial hysterectomy that I had because of endometriosis (in 18 years I have had 17 surgeries for this).

I really need help as I am crying as I write this letter. The pain has gotten so much worse over the two years, that I can not take it anymore. I am taking percocet that does nothing at all, I was actually scared that I might have bone cancer. I had blood work done and everything came back fine so I went to rheumatoid DR who I am not happy with. He tried to tell me that I am extremely double jointed, (I am not sure where he sees this at, I can barely move) and feels that this is part of my problem and also says I have symptoms of Fibro. He put me on trazodone 50mg that I took but is way too strong, I cut it in half and still too strong, it even makes me tremble.

I have suffered with pain since I was fifteen because of the "endometriosis" and still do suffer from it. Now I am not sure I can handle this horrible joint pain, I feel like such a mess, I cant function. It is such an effort for me to leave the house. I am always so dazed and confused. There are days I don't recognize things in my own house that have been there for a long time, and that really scares me.

Thanks for listening.

PJ.

Chapter 5,

How To Almost Have a Bad, Bad Day

Dear World,

Last night I was relaxing in a nice warm bath and started feeling ants crawling on me. I thought "Oh no" not another flare up, give me a break! Then I opened my eyes and ants were crawling on me. I jumped straight up out of the bathtub (not easy for a Fibro) and got them off. I then killed them in the natural way (I'm allergic to bug spray) **bang, bang, splat.** I had a lot of trouble settling down to sleep, I kept feeling antsy. So I dragged myself out of bed this morning, and finished cleaning the kitchen about the time my husband left. So then I go in the bathroom again and didn't notice he had found more ants and he used the spray, **spray, spray, spray**, etc. I was washing up so quickly so I could just get out of there. When I was about to push the button on the deodorant, I realized I was holding the can of ant spray. (The last time I was accidentally sprayed, it took 3 months for the hives and rashes to go away.) He had left the can next to the deodorant so that I would see it and put it away. Well, I still have it. He's out of town right now, but when he gets back tomorrow, I'm going to hit him in the head with the can. **smash, smash, smash.**

V.

How To Almost Have a Bad Bad Day

Dear World,

Okay—I've got one for yea. I figured I'd be lazy and have a frozen pizza for dinner. Kid's gone, it's just me, I have a new book, I figure I'll read until 20/20 comes on tonight.

So when I pull the pizza out of the box, I think to myself "hmph, this must be one of those new kind of pizzas I've seen on TV that have a crust on the top too. Cool." Pop it in the oven, and start my book.

Few minutes later, I go in to check it.

What I find in the oven looks something like a dinosaur sneeze. Cheese is dripping all over, down to the bottom of the oven in strings. I'm still cleaning it and will probably be cleaning it this time tomorrow. **Brain Fog, Brain Fog.**

I just opened the box upside down and thought it was a crust on top pizza!!!!!!!!!!!!!!!

I cant believe I admitted this.

GG.

Here is another almost bad day.

Dear World,

Mine is an experience with pantyhose, if not usable maybe it will bring a chuckle, anyway. I was invited to a very large wedding reception with all the trimmings and setting that would indeed make the bridal magazines drool. Having FM I was reluctant to go due to the 50 pounds I had gained. My wardrobe was mainly down to nightshirts with such cute screen printings as Tiger. The latest one from my son's college, cute phrases than are not cute, you get the picture.

The morning of, I decided to wear a stretch knit skirt with a matching jacket that was long enough to cover the rolls that were caused when I finally did get into a bra. So the elastic of the waistband combined with the rolls from what was produced by bra, made me look like a side show laugh. OK, the first thing was to try to get into the pantyhose from hell. All inspired from the devil himself. After the mental torture of composing the outfit to wear, taking of the bath with fragrant bath gel and shaving I was ready to attempt the battle of getting dressed. Now here, I must say that I am in lots of pain, no sleep, sore, muscle spasms, a deadline of which I already had taken up over an hour to get moving. I picked out the color of pantyhose and prayed I would not get a run in them. I sat on the side of the bed willing them to just hop on me. After wasting another 10 minutes realizing that this was not going to happen, I began the task. Sitting I tried to arrange them on the floor so I could just put one foot in one leg then the other, no this did not work. It was going to take more physical effort on my part. So with the right foot I managed to bring the leg up to meet my hands half way, gotcha! I stood that leg and slowly wiggled enough to get that right leg up over the knee, ut oh, the left leg was just dangling there. What was I to do with a Fibro body that couldn't get that left leg to move up to match the right one, oh no I said to myself. By this time I had already had to lie back down to rest.

Now I am really behind in schedule. Only one thing to do, that is to roll the right leg back down enough to get the left leg in to make them equal. OK, I hurt, I am exhausted, I know why I don't go out anymore than I do. I love my friends whose daughter is getting married and I AM GOING! After struggling I finally have them partially up to the knees. Now I am praying,

Lord, just a little more effort and slow down the clock and please don't let me start a run with my nails that do look good. Prayers are answered. I got them on, thanked the Lord for helping. I got dressed, picked up my daughter and was only a few minutes late of which nobody noticed since there were several hundred people. If you want to know what hell is like having Fibro, then try putting on a pair of pantyhose. I would tell you what the reception was like but that would be another Fibro story.

C.

Dear World,

Guys and gals—I was shown last night how wonderful real laughter is for us. I had been having the weeks from hell with new pain sprouting out all over. I couldn't get comfortable walking, sitting, lying down, standing—you know the feeling. Well, spent last night for about 3 hours in a "reunion" of sorts laughing my head off. It was the best medicine (besides the **pantyhose** described below). When you're down, it's really hard to laugh at even the funniest of situations, movies, etc. So, I guess my body must have been ready for it. Because it just lifted a lot of pain (temporarily, of course) and made me escape the problems for a period of time. I had to force myself to go, even though it was going to be the highlight of my social year (sad, but true). Was feeling miserable, hadn't slept, etc. But, it **really works.** I wish each one of you could have been there to share the laughs and hope that something tickles your funny bone for hours at a time. You'll really feel better!!

Guys, I know you can't appreciate this part, but the women can.

I have been wearing such loose clothing, slacks, etc., which I can get away with in my community for the work I do. I have

been experiencing new pains that come out of nowhere all of a sudden, but then don't go away. By yesterday afternoon when we drove down to Miami to attend the special function, I was limping worse than I have in my entire life for anything (pain in back right hip). Well, I had to get all trussed up for the event— including that dreaded torture chamber known as **pantyhose**!! I can't say "**immediately**" fast enough! The pain was instantaneously gone, and lasted all through the event. Of course, I could hardly eat because the skirt of my suit was so tight due to weight gain. At any rate, we got back to the hotel and I took off the pantyhose and **viola**, the pain returned mildly. I know it will get worse. So, my wonderful mother's answer was "You know, you can get a larger size and then they won't be as tight." **aarrgh**!! **The next size up is "Queen Size."**
K.

Dear World,

My story is not a bad day rather than a bad night. Although funny now. It was not so funny then. I have a cat breeding business in my home and since I have FM I find that cleaning cages is better for me at night or early morning. I usually sleep until 2pm everyday. I have this special cat litter that looks like little white pearls and what you do with it is, run a blow dryer on it and it cleans it instead of throwing it a way. Of course this is after you scoop out the clumps.

So here I was blow drying the buckets of pearl cat litter, when I tripped over the vacuum cleaner, which hit this bucket of bleach water, which then hit the buckets of pearl cat litter. This was a domino effect. As I and it all came down to a crashing hold on the floor I screamed "ooooooh noooooo". The worse than about mixing pearl cat litter and water is that it expands and becomes a huge mess. I was trying to be quite as my husband was sleeping since it was 2am in the morning. He still didn't wake if you can believe that. But you should of seen the mess I had. I also must tell you that I can only use one arm, cause the other one has such a flare in it that it won't work.

So here I am trying with one arm trying to clean this huge mess up and trying to be quite at the same time. Every time I would scoop up one batch of pearls another batch would appear. This went on for hours. So finally I managed to clean it and the rest of the cages about the time it was for my husband to get up. When he finally woke up and stumbled into the kitchen to find me sitting in the chair exhausted. He say's "We really need to clean this kitchen sometime it looks terrible." I thought I would just about hit him in the head. If he only knew what I had been going through. I just turned and looked at him and said "Knock yourself out, I am going to bed. Good night dear." He gave me a kiss and off I went.

PJ.

A prayer from Jan McDonald:

Dear God,

To you, Who created all things, who loves us so much that You would have us live forever, We come boldly before you in prayer. We know that you have borne our infirmities and carried our sorrows on the cross. By your wounds we have been healed. The Bible gives us many examples where you healed people and since you are the same yesterday, today and tomorrow we claim this healing power in our lives today. We claim it for our whole bodies. We ask also that you draw us closer that we may know your character and actually feel your love for us. We thank you ahead of time because we know that you listen and hear our supplication. Like a child who takes his bike to his daddy to be fixed, goes away and plays, knowing that when he returns the job will be done, so we lay our lives in your loving care, knowing the job will be done. In the precious name of Jesus we ask these things and thank you. AMEN.

Chapter 6,

Children with Fibromyalgia

I'm a 15 year old girl, and for the past 8 months I've been living with symptoms similar to those that all the adults seem to have. I've been from doctor to doctor, and no one seems so find anything "physically" wrong with me. All I know is I don't feel good and no one will listen. I don't even have anyone to talk to compare symptoms with. I would like everyone to know that kids have this too. They have to no that we are not all lazy. It is tuff being so young and not being able to do all the things that your friends do. No one seems to understand you because on the outside you look just fine. All my friends think I fake it to get attention. I wish for one day they could feel the way I do. Maybe then they would understand. I think that there should be a message boards on the Internet for kids with Fibromyalgia to talk to other kids with their same problem. I've never met anyone who feels like I do, and I feel basically alone.

Dear world,

My 16 year old daughter was just diagnosed with fibromyalgia. It has been a whirlwind for the past year with her. We have gone to so many doctors and she has been through the mill with tests. Finally all the doctors collaborated and came up with this diagnosis. It's relieving knowing what is wrong with her finally

but as a mother it is so disheartening to know it will be a life long battle for her. I myself suffer from osteoarthritis and fibromyalgia as well. I know it's all too real and my heart goes out to my daughter and anyone of any age who suffers from this horrible condition. There are days when she cannot bring herself to get out of bed and days when she falls asleep in school during class. Unfortunately there is not enough understanding of this disorder so sympathy has been hard to come by from her teachers. Her junior year of high school has been an academic nightmare but frankly I would give anything for her to have her health instead of good grades. I wish I had some advice on how to broach the subject on more understanding to this condition? She gets labeled a hypochondriac. On top of everything before this all came to a head she suffers from severe, debilitating, chronic migraines which over the course of the year have gotten worse. We now have to inject her with immitrex instead of rushing her to the ER. Thank god for immitrex. She also takes an anti-depressant called Paxil. Her neurologist and rhematoligist have come up with a dose to alleviate (or try to) her symptoms. They want her to start taking PT to loosen her muscle and joints. The thought of exercise makes her sick to her stomach for she can barely move about on so many days. I feel for all of us!!
D.

Dear World,

Okay, I'm not going to sleep if I don't get this off my mind. After two years of denying and excuses I finally took my daughter to see the pediatrician in order to rule out any other possibilities besides Fibro. I am afraid for her because of the pains, fatigue, and neuro symptoms she has been having. It went as I expected—The doctor doesn't believe in FM and thinks we are just making ourselves sick. Don't worry, I definitely stood up for us Fibromites! She said children do not get FM. I said yes they do and they have pediatric sections in books on FM. She said she hasn't seen any in her 15 years of practice and I said "maybe you have now, and you are probably going to see increasing numbers of us." She's checking out blood work for juvenile arthritis, x-rays for her knees, endometriosis, migraines and such. Does this sound familiar people? She has no problem with giving me a referral (if I need one)to a rheumy. She had one in particular to set up an appointment with. I said I knew where she stood "You don't believe in Fibro and I want a rheumy that specializes in Fibro" At the end of the appointment she told my daughter very strongly "You do not have Fibromyalgia!" She also requested to speak to my daughter alone. While in private she asked if my husband and I fight, if her and I fight, if she was happy. My daughter told her every-thing was fine and she was happy. Then the doctor told her that this was all in her head and she needed to be happy. Ha! My daughter already knew that the reason we haven't taken her in sooner was because they were going to blame her being sick on either the parents or the "controlling child." Their solution is to run tests (which was why I was there to make sure nothing else was causing this), and give her sleeping pills because she's not sleeping well(which should also help with the headaches). She is also being sent to a neurologists for the headaches. They are also taking stool samples because of the stomach problems. So I guess we will be able to rule out everything in a short period of time. The problem is trying to find a rheumy that believes in Fibro who will see a 13 year old. They usually won't see children at-least the ones I know. I fear I will not be able to find a pedi-atric rheumy that believes in this illness. The fact is, and I told the pediatrician, that whether she believes in my daughters symptoms or not—doesn't change the fact that they exist! I told her that Fibro was real whether she believes in it or not. We agreed to disagree. What a shame! Here's a woman who could help children that are hurting but instead has chosen to invalidate their suffering. Maybe the sleeping pills will ease her symptoms. It's a long shot but it is a possibility. I mean, who in their right mind would want this for their child!?! Give me a break! She had these symptoms before I even knew I had Fibro and that my symptoms were related and not separate entities. My symptoms have been documented for years without me having any knowledge of a disease like Fibro. I guess all we Fibromites decided to conjure up these odd symptoms so we could fake an epidemic. We are pretty amazing because we did this without knowing each other or each others doctors. Aren't we devious to do this to the medical community!?! LOL!!! There! I feel better!! Good night!

And for us who know it is real......

Fibro Hugs!

A.

Dear World,

Hi! I am almost in tears. I am 14 years old and I felt like I was all alone going through these terrible symptoms until I found a Internet site for people with Fibromyalgia. I thought if I read about some other people it might help. It has helped in one way but it also made me feel bad for all the others too. I have had this for about 4 years now. I have gone through 3 MRI's and a bone scan. I love playing sports, but I had to quit everything because of the pain. I tried to play soft ball this last summer because I felt better, but I ended up quitting it after the first few games. To all the kids out there—I hope we are feel better soon. This is a real drag to have this happen to us.

J.

Dear World,

It must be frustrating having to deal with insensitive teachers. I have copied information for each of my daughter's teachers, plus spoken one on one with each one of them. Some seem more understanding than others. My 13 year old daughter has had FM for almost two years. We have come a long way.

She has had a flare up about every couple of months since she was first diagnosed. My daughter started PT about a month after she was diagnosed. At first it seemed like she hurt more after PT, but as the time went by we found out just how weak she really was. Because she was weak she was getting hurt much more frequently. She also built up her stamina. (she didn't have much in the beginning) She has been through PT four times. But the last time she got hurt, we started to massage her right away and exercised with her and we didn't have to go through PT. She does low impact sports, swimming and bike riding and walking. She does not run. She feels the best when she takes a bath in the morning and does stretching exercises. She loves school and works really hard to keep up with her friends. Her best support is our church youth group.

J.

Dear World,

My daughter was diagnosed in Jan after approx. 18 mos. of symptoms. With many doctors and tests. She, too, is in her junior year of high school. She was out of school for 5 months

on home instruction, and has just gotten back but on a shortened day. If you get documentation from your doctors as to her diagnosis and associated symptoms, your daughter is guaranteed certain academic accommodations under section 504 of the disability act. I have been fighting to get my daughter classified as handicapped by her school but my district is reluctant. However, they did offer me accommodations which include: home instruction as needed for MD documented flare-ups when attendance is possible, a shortened day (currently my daughter only goes in for 4 periods and gets home tutored on the others) as needed per MD documentation when fatigue and pain make it impossible to tolerate a full day of school. If your school has a policy that drops kids for a certain amount of absences, that policy must be waived if the absences are associated with her condition. Also within the school setting—an elevator pass and extra passing time between class. Maybe a book buddy to help carry her load and a second set of books at home. Extra time to complete assignments especially ones that require a lot of typing or writing (due to wrist and joint pain), and gym as tolerated with no long distance running. The shortened day was really a blessing for us. She would go for a day or two then be totally Zonked, exhausted and unable to concentrate or go to school for a day or two. Being able to sleep a little later and come home early has worked very well for her, and it also enables her to get some social interaction in at school. Five months home was getting very depressing to her. Go to the school with doctor's notes asking for these accommodations, and any others that you think may make her life easier. By law they must give them to her.
H.

Dear World,

Hi! I am 12 years old! I have been diagnosed two or three years ago! I have been going to doctors' years before then. I have went to all different types of doctors. Just name any kind and I've been there! I had a lot of doctors tell me right to my face that it is all in my mind or head or even I'm faking it! I would never ever fake something so terrible!

I have been in a wheelchair for a while and I can't take it! It feels like knifes going into my legs every second of the day! That's how it is for me. Maybe there is another young person out there who feels the same. If so, see your not alone. Just hang in there, I am.
M.

Dear World.

I'm from Jasper, In. I am 16 years old, my birthday is Feb.20, 1984. I've been sick my whole life, but last year my legs, hands, feet were hurting really bad. I was missing a lot of school too. The nurse at school said that I needed to go see my family doctor. He did a lot of blood test and X-rays. He found out that one of the arthritis test was high. So he sent me to a Children's Hospital to see a joint doctor. She found out that I have Chronic Fatigue Syndrome and FM. But when I had flair's my parents couldn't take off work and take me to the hospital that is three hours away. So we found a joint doctor closer by which is just one hour away. So he did a lot of blood test and found out I have lupus now. Also during this time I've had really bad menstrual problems, so heavy and stuff. So my mom took me to see a OBGYN and he did a probe ultrasound and found a floating cyst and endometriosis. So I have to take Lupron shots which makes me even feel worse. Also when I was 15 I had a

cyst in my breast. They did thyroid test and found it was low one time, but didn't do anything , because it was fine the next time. Also I have asthma, Bladder problems, Stomach problems, Colon problems, and allergies. It's no fair! I use to be a dancer, and a gymnast. They want to send me to Mayo Clinic. But insurance will not pay. It has been really bad money wise. We go to this doctor and he says this and the next one says that. I'm so tried of being sick!!
J.

Dear World,

If you are thinking of getting pregnant I would like to lend some advice I have on the subject. I have Fibromyalgia. Although, I have never been pregnant I have worked with pregnant woman who are afraid of delivery, etc. I would, of course, recommend things you already know like teaching your patient meditation techniques incorporated with a form of trance. The earlier she starts learning these techniques the less fear she'll have when she goes into labor. I have found that music that the woman find enjoyable is helpful. Encourage her to talk about her fears. Make sure the people who will be helping her know, in advance, about her FMS status, especially the anesthesiologist. I would go with her to talk to the Chief of Anesthesiology to find out if he and his staff have ever dealt with such a case and she can find out ahead of time what they can do for her to deal with her pain more efficiently. I would recommend that she doesn't wait until she is in agony before she has pain relief. Go with her to the place she will be delivering at and discuss her concerns and make sure she has a plan in place for when she delivers and for when she comes home so she is not overwhelmed by the situation immediately. The last advice I can give you as an FMS

patient is that while FMS may go on forever, Labor and Delivery will end. I don't know if any of this is helpful, but I hope so. Good luck and Best wishes,
P.

Dear World,

I am so sorry. It is so tough parenting a Fibro teen. I know what they mean when they say you'd rather they have their health. Some mornings I just walk out of my 14 year old daughter's room and cry. I could never let her see how much affect this syndrome is having on her father and me. She too has horrible days that she can't even sit up in bed unassisted. My daughter is currently on 500mg of Naprosyn (pain medication)/2x's a day and 10 mg of Ambien (sleep medication) then she takes 800 mg of ibuprofen as needed. My daughter also suffers from severe migraines. I just hate it all!! No one understands unless they've been in our place. I have to force my daughter to move, to walk, to stretch…in order to keep her muscles mobile. When she was first diagnosed she had been bedridden with pain for 4 months and when the rheumatologist said she had to start "exercising"…she cried. But, it really helped!! Just a 10 minute walk a day makes all the difference in the world. Good luck!!

Dear World,

I am a 35 year old female with FM and I feel my 5 year old daughter has it. I am getting ready to go purchase some "specific" vitamins and herbs to help her. I truly believe that with Fm you have to do at least a few different things to help yourself. I started sleeping on a magnetic mattress pad about a ½ hears ago. It has helped me to fall asleep and now I lay down I maybe in pan when I lay down but with in a much shorter amount of time I fall asleep. I seem to sleep deeply. I find myself waking up in the morning in the same position I fell asleep in. This has never happened before. I was always up every couple of hours. My daughter was 4 when I put her on a magnetic mattress pad and she started immediately sleeping through the night. It is just one of the things that will help. Especially if you are having trouble sleeping. Sleep is such a key to our health. So are many other things in life. We all need the deep R.E.M sleep because that is when our body repairs itself. It may seem overwhelming at times but just remember you can get through it. just take one step at a time.

S.

Dear World,

My daughter age 16 was diagnosed in January. Her biggest problems are fatigue and mental fog; the pain is secondary right now. She was put on Elavil 20 mg at night for increased restorative sleep. It didn't help and depression developed. (I'm not sure if it is because of the sleeplessness or her condition). We cut the Elavil and went to a psychiatrist (her rheumatologist does not prescribe anything else but Elavil because she feels a psychiatrist should control those meds). He gave her a sleeper— Sonata, and Zoloft to begin at 25mg and increase to 100. (she weighs 175 lb.). She has been restless and poorly sleeping ever since (5 days now). I called the psychiatrist who suggested take the Zoloft in the morning, and the sleeper at night and she can take 2 if necessary. He said that sleeplessness is also a symptom of depression and once that is under control, she should sleep better. My daughter says he is crazy, all she needs is a good few night's sleep. She does not want to take any anti-depressants saying she is ill, not depressed. Meanwhile, she cries, complains, lays around, etc. I am at a loss. Which is causing which? Which should be treated? I read about others who are treated with antidepressants. Is this for depression or for increased sleep? Do the two go hand in hand? Finally, how can I help my daughter through this? I am trying to be supportive but I asked her to try it the way the doctor asked for 1 more week and she thought I was betraying her. This is just a touch of what we go through every day of our lives.

Best Wishes

W.

Dear World,

I was not sleeping as well after several years on Ambient. My rheumatologist switched me to Sonata and I had 2 of the most awful nights of my life. I never went fully to sleep. A million thoughts raced through my mind all night and I was too tired to get up. After 2 nights I called him and he just upped the dosage of ambient and I am fine again. One of the biggest hurdles to overcome with Fibro is learning what works and what doesn't with **your** body. At least as an adult I felt in charge of what we were trying and could say when it was enough. At a young persons age they should be listened to. Tell them that the antidepressant is not for depression. They are seratonin reuptake inhibitors. Seratonin is the feel good substance most people's brains make and send through their bodies through the spinal fluid and out through the blood stream. It blocks pain and the feelings of depression.

In Fibro patients it is not used in the correct way and is taken back before it does any good. So you need a reuptake inhibitor. This is a very unprofessional way to explain it but there is a world of information about it available. The best thing your daughter or son can do is to start reading about all this and learn what is available. Ask your Doctor to let you try it and see what works best. No one can tell you what is working and you won't get better if you sit back to see what the Doctor can do to fix you. If you wait for some one to come riding up on a white horse to save you, you will be very sick for a long time. This has got to be a partnership with the very best doctor you can find. Why in the world would a rheumatologist send them to a phyc? For help? Is he one of those "this is all in your head" Doctors? I sure hope not as I thought we old ladies that have had it for years would be the last generation to have to deal with that. If they are truly depressed due to their illness and the helplessness that is one thing, but don't ever let anyone make them think this is anything but a physical illness.

I always knew I was different and carried a lot of guilt, that if I could just buck up like others I would be fine. I thought I was lazy because I was told that as a kid when I was just too tired to move. This is an awful burden for a kid to carry. When I wasn't flaring I was a ball of fire and I ;have always been an over achiever if anything yet I felt I was still not as good as others as I could never maintain because another flare would come and I was in the dumps again. When I say "we feel your pain" I am not joking. We learn so much by sharing. My 13 year old grand-daughter has just came through her 1st flare and she is the 5th generation to have this as far back as I know.
M.

Dear World,

I live in Georgia and I don't have any family here beside my son. Once I showed him an article about Fibro, his whole attitude changed. However, my mom came down to help me. I had a serious flare up in March. I'm back at work for 4-6 hours a day (some days). Of course, there are some days that are better than others. Of course, my mom did not see the worse of it. However, I must have been complaining about my pain or stiffness or moaning. She said, you are draining my strength. I was really hurt by that but then I remembered the board and the posts that said "people don't understand." I told her if you think I'm draining your strength now, I'm glad you didn't come down here when I was bedridden. Here, I thought I was doing really good. I went to the store with her and said I can not stay too long. After being in the store on my feet for 1/2 hour, I said Mom, its time to go. After telling her this three times, with a span of about 5-10 minutes each, I left her in the store and sat on the bench. Then I was fussed at about leaving her in the store. I thank God for my mom but I wish she could understand…I did tell her that she was here so I could drain her strength…we both laughed at that one.

A prayer from Jan McDonald:

For children-Daddy God, I know how much you love me and I don't understand why I don't feel good. In the story of Joseph, his brothers did those bad things to him (Gen 37) and you turned it to good. Since you are always the same, I believe that you will do that for me. I believe that you will also make my life good, like Joseph. I trust you, Daddy God, and thank you. I ask these things in Jesus name, AMEN.

Chapter 7,

Wonderful husbands

Dear World,

I am a 28 years old. I am married to the most wonderful husband anyone could ask for. I was diagnosed with Fibro. on August,1999. I got married on August 21,1999. I was a hairdresser for this company for over 4 yrs. They fired me but, I am going to fight it because people need to realize that just because I have Fibro. and Hypoglycemia that I am not a week doll that needs special attention every day of my life. When I have good days I do everything that I can because I know that I will have bad months. I use to work 8 to 9 hours. a day and I would go to Martial Arts for a couple of hours. Come home and clean up. Now I had to quit, but I still read and keep up with it that way. I am very proud of myself when I can clean the kitchen by myself. I have been on Zoloft,Clonapam,Prozac,2 800 mg of IBprorin twice a day Dolgic for migraines, Vistaril, and Celebex 200 mg. None of it has helped me at all. I do not like to depend on medication. Sometimes I wake up out of a dead sleep because the pain hurts so bad that I wake up screaming and crying. I have a wonderful doctor. I do recommend my specialist because I know more about Fibro. than she does and she is supposed to be a specialist. My vision comes and goes. The aches and pain alone would keep me up. I have Insomnia. I

cannot be out in direct sunlight and my memory is getting terrible. My husband is always there for me. For Christmas, I was so sick that I could not get up. Even though I was in pain and I could not even keep my head up. My husband picked me up and carried me outside so that I could see our lights. That was our First Christmas together being married. We have been together for almost 8 years, through all of my bad days, pain, crying, and cannot remember things. My husband has been there for me, no matter how much I cry and nothing seems to go right for us. He is always there for me. I was fired from my job this year, but we will fight together. Keep happy thoughts and memories. My great-grandmother is 99 years. old and she is in better shape than me.(HA HA) I look at life through her eyes now. Live for the minute not the day. Try to keep a good thought if possible.
S.

Dear World,

Let me tell you about my wonderful husband. I have been married only 6 years and every since we got married I got sick. He has stuck by me through thick and thin. Once we found out what I had and what life was going to be like, he just jumped in with both feet. My husband works 80 hours a week at his job then comes home and takes care of me. Not to say I do nothing. I try to get as much as I can get done and he just helps to finish. Some times I come home and he will get off early and he will have cleaned the whole kitchen so I don't have to. Or maybe he will do the laundry or help me fold it. If I ask him to do something for me it's no problem. He just does it. He always rubs me and gives me vibration massages. He constantly asks me how I am and if there is anything he can do to make me

more comfortable. He even lets me rest when I need to. I really can't say enough about him. He is every women's dream only he is all mine.
Author.

Dear World,

My husband is wonderful. He never complains and listens when I complain which sometimes seems like all the time. When I can't cook, he does. Whenever I don't feel like going somewhere, he stays with me. When I say "help," he says "how." I am truly blessed.
V.

Dear World,

My story that I have to tell begins with my husband and friends. Even my family would just look at me when I would say I was in pain, over and over, and would say things like "if you would kept going from doctor to doctor you'll get better. I think he was just fed up because I couldn't do things as before and would complain wish the pain and trying different meds and going through the side affects. Well, one night he was sitting next to me at the computer waiting to go on line. I had been telling him about the Fibro board I found and about how I wasn't the only one with this pain. I think he thought oh well. Well, I said read this. He started reading this board and so happen that night everyone was talking about their pain and symptoms and they were just like mine, after he read this board, I saw a difference in him. He is behind me all the way. It is not in my head now he knows this is for real. He knows there are more people out there like me. So having my husband read the board helped me so much. If you have trouble with the people you care about, have them read a Fibro message board. You might be surprised the difference it will make.

P.

Dear World,

I have for many years been undiagnosed with Fibromyalgia. I finally, three years ago got the answer I needed. My husband has read a few parts of a good book on Fibromyalgia. He understands so much you won't believe it. He started a business for me so I could just work part time and even on the 2 days I do work, if I don't feel well, he will fill in for me. It happened this weekend. He won't let me over do it, although I am guilty as heck. He is so good with me and gives me support always. He is the most wonderful husband in the world. I couldn't ask for better.

G.

Dear World,

Last night my hubby and I were talking. I told him the pain would get much worse. Even that I would eventually have to have pain medication. He understood this and I told him I didn't want to be a burden to him and he told me he would take care of me as long as he could. Then we would have to figure something out when he could no longer. he's very loving and caring and supportive to me. I don't know what I would do without him.

C.

Dear World,

My husband is wonderful not because I have FMS but because he learned how to be a good man from positive influences in his family consisting of 3 women and 1 man. From the get go, he was led down the road of compassion due to his mom's and sister's health problems at various times.

He was encouraged to try all things, good and bad and see the differences. He has done both and has developed an all around personality. He is not prejudice. Why is this important? The answer is because prejudice comes in all forms, not just colors, creeds and ethnaticities. He understands that though I'm not physically what I once was, he sees that spiritually and mentally I am the **same** and will always be. Because he sees that, he sees my pain more than many even try. He took me to the ER one week 4 times. Recently, 2 times within three days I have went to the ER. I sit here thinking I might have to go again tonight. Why doesn't he complain? He sees me vomit from pain. He sees my blood pressure go skyward from pain. He sees the raccoon eyes I've developed. He has seen me get needles shoved into me bigger than he would allow. He's sees me every day get out of bed and keep on trying to fight this no matter how much or how little I do. Even when I'm not able physically, I am with him in other ways.

He will cook if needed but I do it for relaxation. He will clean if I'm not OCDing at that moment. He will go to the pharmacy anytime, day or night on or off the job for my meds. He will walk out of his job within an hour to get me to where I need to be for medical treatment. The list goes on but he tells me the most impressive thing is this: I remain a mother of two children who need me and one who has a horrible mental illness. I remain a wife in spite of pain in all ways. And I'm always his friend ready to listen even if I'm too tired to respond.

My husband is terrific because he sees me seeing myself trying to quit physically when mentally I won't allow it. He attends **every** doctor's appointment with me. He goes to every school meeting regarding my son to make sure I'm okay and to take notes on foggy days. He brings me coffee every morning and has for almost four years. He gives me the little things that mean the most and that makes him wonderful. He doesn't make me feel guilty about my illness and I don't bore him with repetitive information. However, he will always listen to anything new I find. He pushes the doctors as much as I do.

Oh what a subject. I could go on longer but I think I'll stop with this: He is wonderful because he is my friend and friends don't let each other down no matter how tough it gets.

Dear World,

To the persons who don't have husbands to rely on in hard times, I am so sorry. I thought that is what love was. I never for an instant thought my husband would not understand. He works and helps me with house work. I couldn't ask for a better man. Above all that after 12 years, I still have to beat him off me with a stick. I guess I am extremely blessed. I just couldn't imagine going through this alone. Today, Sunday, I had a bad day. My husband went and got us something to eat at a restaurant. Then he straightened up the house and did the dishes as I took a much needed nap. When I got up, he gave me a message. He fed all our animals and cut the grass. He is always by my side through thick and thin. I love him with all my heart and soul. I've made it through another day with love from friends with no faces.

Dear World,

Well, My hubby is good in the way that he has tolerated my pain,depression,anxiety,17 surgeries, no children, lack of sex, menopause, and now the Fibro. He really is soooo distracted and if one thing goes wrong in his world boy, do we all know about it. He thinks, "I will take care of it." I cant say much because I don't work now. He works a tight schedule and I don't. Just wish he would look at me when I talk, but I know he cares we have been together forever. H.

Dear World,

Last night the fatigue hit me like a truck. Perhaps it the underlying stress of my big day tomorrow or maybe it's the dreary weather. My husband tells me he can usually see it in my face. I look very drained and flushed. He was a sweetheart so we ate out and he folded the laundry I had washed & dryer dried during the day, when we got home. I went to bed about 8:30 and was probably asleep a little after 9pm. I was up a few times during the night thanks to my overactive bladder. I feel like I'm ready for a nap. My eyes are so heavy.
O.

Chapter 8,

How Fibromyalgia effects our sex life

Dear World,

I would like to complain about fribro and sex. Can you say "major hip cramping" if it's not over in under 10 minutes I can count on major, major hip pain for the next couple of days, not to mention increased neck, back, and groin pain. I used to be active and love sex, now I almost run away from it. I hate the effects it has on my life. I call it the after math. I wish I could enjoy it again if not for my sake for my husband sake. Thank god he doesn't know it is really that bad. He knows it hurts but I would never tell him that it was that bad. He is a good man and I don't want to disapoint him. Thanks for listening.
H.

Dear World,
OUCH,

That name is so fitting for the subject. My hips feel like cold cement bricks. My knees and his are both shot. I have Spinal Stenosis (back) so I sure can relate. As for the groin pain, I also experience that and thought I was the only one. Migraines, sharp shooting pains in my breast, tightness of my chest, numbness and tingling of my neck, down to my feet. I have also had numbness in my tongue and was told to tell the doctor about that because it means something. Sex, those were the days…God Bless Him for putting up with me but I have to be creative. LOL…good luck, your not alone.

Z.

Dear world,

My hips and pelvic area are always hurting. I'm use to it now. Sex can be painful. But there are many things you can do.

1. Eat a can of smoked oysters the night before. Stimulates feeling.
2. Use candles and music.
3. Have a special meal in the bedroom and share thoughts.

There is SO much more to intimacy than intercourse. I know it's our desired goal, but if we focus on the other person and time with him with (her) the end result may be less strained and come more naturally and easily. My husband and I have been married for 10 yrs and 9 mo. and our private life has changed just as much as our public life. But we still love each other. Probably more now than 11 yrs ago. Sex is a rarity. When it does occur, it is very special to both of us and gets us through until the next time.

P.

Dear World,

I found out my husband was reluctant to initiate anything because he thought I hurt too much and didn't want me to feel worse or obligated. We really talked about it and now he realizes that I need him just as much when I am hurting. As a matter of fact, I find a good romp will do wonders! Must mean all those endomorphs or something! So talk openly and things might heat up for you too.

W.

Dear world,

I can certainly relate......however a position I have found that doesn't hurt is side lying with him behind also on your tummy. Another thing I try to do is have everything done and rest before he comes home. I will be 50 in August and our sex life is great. No we do not have the luxury of some postions but where there is a will there is a way.

I think sex is very important to us, to provide the intimacy and enhance our womanly feelings. We were just married in April and I am having the worst symptoms of my 25 yrs with this disease. Some days are spent in bed period. So don't give up there is sex with fibro just as there is life with fibro, maybe not someone elses idea of life but I am living one day at a time (sometimes one hour at a time)

W.

Dear World,

I have the same problem. I just turned 45 and have no sex desire. This is killing my husband. I stay so tired, and hurt so much I just can't stand for anyone to touch me. My dr. gave me hormone shots, but they didn't help either. I take effexor and Klonapin, so I figure the Med. have alot to do with it also.

T.

Dear World,

My problem is, the medicain I take (paxil) I often forget about sex. I go all month long and maybe if I am lucky I might get a little excited towards the end. If I go off the medicain then I am a horrible person. Trust me it is better to take it then to not. However I try to keep track of when we last did it so I don't leave my poor husband unatended to. I can usaully tell when I start to hear him make sugetions to me like "Your looking good today". Then I phsyc myself up and let him have it. Sometimes it feels good and I can get into it, but most of the time I just fake it. As long as he feels good that's the main thing. I know this probably sounds terrible. But my mom always said if you can keep a man happy in the bedroom and in the kitchen then you will never loose him. Well I don't know if it true but I have been married for 26 years so there must be something to it.

M.

Dear World,

I used to wiegh 115 pounds and considered myself pretty frisky. Now that I have Fibromyalgia, I have gained 130 more pounds. Now I wiegh 245. It has made me miserable when it comes to sex. I have to do it differently because it is so uncomfortable. I just don't feel sexy anymore. I have tried every diet I can think of, but nothing seems to work. Well I guess I will keep trying.

R.

Chapter 9,

My Story

A note from the writer: I was once alone and didn't know where to turn so I hope this helps another person who feels they are in the same position.
  Gentle hugs Dawna

Dear World,

  I would like to begin by telling you my story from the earliest that I can remember. In the summer of 1975 I was 9 years old. We had a great big in ground pool and all summer long I played with my friends swimming everyday. I was a typical kid completely healthy. One morning I was really tired so I slept in. My mom thought I was just tired from playing day after day so hard. But that day I never got out of bed. I would wake up for a little while but for the most part I sleeped for about 3 days. On the 3rd day my mom got so worried, she took me to a doctor that was also a friend of hers. I remember driving a 3 hr drive in which I slept all the way down there. She had me tested for diabetes. They thought because I was sleeping so much that that's what it had to be. Well it wasn't, the doctor said I was just a exhausted kid and that I would snap out of it a few days after I got some rest. I guess I did cause that's the last time I did that for a long time. I still can remember that I was always somewhat tired but not enough to notice if it was any-more tired than anyone else.

The next part of my life growing up through my teenage years and my young adult life was a lot of a blur, because for one I didn't really pay much attention to how I was feeling. I did party a lot and was out all hours and led a very fast paste life so like I said the most I can remember about it is that I was always real emotional. I was always crying over some boyfriend.Who knows if the way I led my life has anything to do with this or not.

The next thing that I can really remember was when I was about 27 years old I started sleeping after work and sometimes I would sleep from 4:30 in the afternoon until the next day at 6:00 am when I had to get up and go back to work. I went to the doctor for the first time in a long time and he just told me that I was probably not getting to the REM state at night and gave me some sleeping pills to take.Well I started taking them and at first was more sleeper than ever. I then decided I didn't like the way they made me feel so I quit them and started an exercise program. I thought maybe it would make me sleepy at night and I would sleep good. Well I guess I got better at least I stopped sleeping after work. Looking back at this I know now it had to be depression. I just didn't know it then. I was in a bad relationship and a very stressful job, but I was so use to having my life in such a mess that it was normal for me. Maybe sleep-ing all the time was my only excape from my day to day crap I had to deal with. I do know that things did get better when I stopped my relationship with my old boyfriend and I started a new one with my now current husband who by the way is absultly the best. So now that my life is great I shouldn't have anymore problems right? Wrong.

After we were married we were forced to move because the place we were renting was being sold. We looked and looked and then finally decided to move into my moms house. I knew in my heart it wasn't the right thing to do. I had done that before and even though I was against it we did it anyway.

My mom is a very wonderful person and there is no one in the world I would rather have for a mother than her. She would do anything in the world for me and I would for her. But with both of us being so sick and not knowing what was happening to each other we had a hard time dealing with it. Looking back I know now that if I or her had not been sick one of us would of took care of the other and the situation would of been a great one. Now once again we live a part and we are the best friends we have alway been.

We spent a year in one of the rooms in my moms house. She had problems of her own that she was dealing with and I was having a hard time handling it. I didn't know it then but she was as sick as I was. I don't think she even knew it. I also was working on a new business with the hopes that I would start this great business that would take me out of the current stressful situation. Anyway I was working around the clock. I was dealling with my mom and trying to do what she wanted reguarding fixing the house up, working my job and trying to get my new business off the ground.

One morning while getting ready for work I had gotten out to the shower and wrapped a towel around my head. I then went to pull a T-shirt on over my head with the towel still on it and it snapped my head forward. I thought I would see stars. The pain was so excrusiating. I screamed for my husband. He took me to my primary doctor. When he finaly saw me he couldn't tell me why this happened just that it was no big deal. Sure not for him. He gave me a shot of cortisone in my neck and from there I was able to lift it half way. He sent me home with pain killers. I then went to see a massage theropist. He could hardly put his hands on me for the pain was so great. It took about a week and a half before I could lift my head up all the way. He said that I just stress out all my ligaments and I was so out of alinement. I then spent 5 months in theropy for my neck and shoulders and arms. It finaly got to a point when I thought I was back to normal again. Needless to say my business I started well it went down the tubes. And as for living at my moms well we bought a house for ourself and moved out. So now things looked pretty good again. Until the summer of 1996.

I was planning a birthday party for my wonderful husband. Before the guests arrived I wanted to spruce the place up so of course I was busy doing house chores just like everyone does. I was almost done when I went into my bathroom and noticed my tub was dirty, so I had some cleaner handy and I sprayed the tub and like a dummy I just used my hands to wipe out the tub not thinking it would hurt anything. Afterward I notice my hands where a little funny feeling like extra clean or numb. Well I thought it would go away. It didn't. It only got worse. I really almost couldn't feel the palms of my hands they were so numb and tingly. I went back to the massage therepist because I has such great luck with him in the past. But even he couldn't get my hands back to normal. So I thought OK now you have got Carpal Tunnel so off to the doctor I went.

I went to a specialist who said no you don't have that. He thought I had some type of nerve damage. Well then I went to a neurologist and by the time I went to see him more systems started. I would bend my neck forward and my spine would go numb and tingle down to my feet. Well I went to see him and when I told him about my spine going numb and my feet going numb, he told me he wanted me to go to the hospital right away because he thought that I had a shifting spine and wanted to do surgery right away. I was in pure shock. I was crying and I called my husband and we went to the hospital where they took these real intense exrays and found nothing wrong. Thank God because the specialist told me that it was a matter of time and I would be a Christopher Reed.

Well he was wrong.Still I had the numbness and I started to get real tired and started to ache everywhere. I could hardly move. So from there I went to see my primary doctor again and he said "well lets try this specialist who works with MS patients". So I went there for more tests.Yea know buy this time I have had so many blood tests done that I thought I didn't have any blood left. Anyway I went through a MRI which is a brain scan or body scan exray and when we went back to the specialist for the results. He said "that he thought I was 90 percent sure that I had MS. Well I just said no way. There is no real proof and I just don't think so. Anyway if I did what could they do to help me. "Nothing" he said, I wasn't bad enough. Well I went back to my primary doctor again who said I am sending you to a Arthritis specialist. And if he doesn't find something then he said he would send me to the Mayo clinic in Portland because he just couldn't figure out what else to do.

Well I went and after a few more blood tests and he did this exam where he pushed on my back and arms and legs and because I had all these tender spots he said you have Fibromyalgia. I said what is that? And will I die from it? He said no you won't die from it you will only feel like you will die from it. He went and got a pamphlet to help explain it to me. They haven't don't much research on it so trying to help people with it is hard. He started me on Ultram for the pain and for a boost out of fatigue and then some sleeping drugs to help me sleep. He told me that one of the reasons I felt bad is that I probably haven't slept in over 15 years. Not to the R.E.M. state anyway.

Over the next year or so I seem to get better just because I knew I wasn't going to die. The medicines I took really took me up and down emotionally. I tried to rest and after a pretty good summer of feeling a little better I went in to turn spin. I started feeling worse and worse. I had to sleep every day at lunch and then from the time I got home at 4:15 to 6:30 every night then make dinner and back in bed at 8 P.M. I sill couldn't get enough sleep. I sleeped all weekend too. I was barley surviving. Sometimes I would be driving home and not only could I not wait to get home to go to bed but sometimes I would almost fall asleep at the wheel. My back would hurt constinly and I was very irritable because of the pain I was in. I would get my sentences mixed up and my speach sometimes wouldn't even make since. I was loosing my hair by the handfuls. I would get hot all of a sudden for no reason or very ice cold and once I was cold I would have to take a hot bath in order to get warm again. My muscles would get so stiff and sometimes I couldn't even hardly move. I was so weak. I walked like a 90 year old women. I felt like one too. My vision would go in an out of focas. My husband did all the house work and to tell you the truth I can't even remember most of it. I tried to stand and do laundry and every 5 minutes I would have to lay down. My head would spin every day and I felt light headed. My body hurt so bad that my husband would use a vibrator on my body to help loosen it up. I finally went to the arthritis specialist again and he said the reason I was so tired is that I had depression. He put me on Paxil which is a anti-depresent. I couldn't imagine that I had depression cause I didn't want to kill myself. I thought if you had depression that that's what you wanted to do. Well he was right I did have depression.

You see depression is a illness not like you think. It can effect so many parts of your body. Now that I look back at my life and my family history I can see that depression runs in my family and maybe I have had it all my life. My grandmother was in a mental institution after trying to kill her self for about 10 years. This was way before I knew her and no one knows to this day why or how she even got better. I have also seen my mother grow through many situations in her life that when I look at them she has depression too. Now later in her life she has many of the same symptoms that I have. Depression causes fatigue and from that everything thing goes to hell. I think that Fibro stems from depression or at least go hand and hand with it. When I was diagnosed with depression I didn't even know I had it. But if you cry at every thing and maybe you are tired all the time you should be checked it doesn't mean you want to end your life. It can sneak up on you with out you even knowing it.

Now for the good news after struggling with this for so long. Now being 4 years. I met a women who is now a very dear friend she has literally saved my life. She and I had become friends from a business venture that I was trying to do and she had seen me falling apart day after day. She one night sat me down and said listen I know you don't believe in herbs, minerals and vitamins but there is this stuff that I have been involved with and it is like nothing on the market that you have ever seen. It was a nurtraint substance that helps rebuild the immune system. Well the expense of it plus I just couldn't believe it would work lead me to tell her maybe someday I would try it but I really didn't believe it. Now you see, the past 6 months that I had been gradually going down hill. I had been seeing a Fibro specialist so they say and everyone of my doctors including the primary kept saying take this vitamins or this herb and all there patients got better, well ha. I tried them and nothing worked. I even tired special diets. I can't truly say I was faithful cause I was looking for immediate results and I didn't get them so they didn't work.

Well my friend said finally that she was going to give me this stuff and that if it worked great if not OK. Well since I wasn't paying for it and she was insisting I tried it. I tried it. Well I can't say that I got immediate results but the information she gave me on the products really made since. So after a month went by I did notice I felt better but my husband and I thought well it is just some remission. I steadily got better every day. So I bought another months supply. Well it saved my life. I really did try the drugs and stuff the doctors gave me and I have to say this is the only thing that has really worked. It is slow but it is kind of like when you get fat you can't loose it all in one day you take time to put it on so it takes time to take it off. I tried to go 2 weeks with out it and I started slipping back into my coma state so I know it works. I have seen others take it too and they too got better. Now it is not a cure all but I think they are on to something. That's where I think our sickness lies. If we can repair or help our immune system get better we have a better chance of feeling better. There are many sources out there and I have listed them in this book so you can try what ever you want. Yes I am byest about the products I take but being fair, I just want you to know don't stop trying things that are out there because one of them might be what your body needs and can help you. I do truly believe that the products I take will help anyone who wants help. But it is up to you.

Even though I don't take any of the prescription drugs anymore and I was feeling much better I thought that there still has to be more to this desease. After being on the natural products for a year, some of my symtoms where comming back little by little. The only way to keep up with it was to take more and more natural products and I thought there just has to be something else. The natural stuff really did help the pain, infact I almost never had any, but my head was still swimming. So I started looking into the Guiafenesin treatment. I have been on that now for about 1 month the dizziness or swimming is getting much better but the pain has come back like a vengences.

They tell me that pain is a good thing. If you hurt badly then you no it is working. The idea behind that, is if it took a while to bring on this disease and it hurt going in, it is going to hurt comming out. Well I am willing to go through the pain if it means in time I will be better for real. I just want to live the life that I was meant to live. We all know what I am talking about.

So if you are out there and you don't feel good and you don't know what to do, I hope that by reading my story it might bring some hope or understanding on what you are going through. Maybe one of the ideas in this book will help you find what makes you feel better. I would try anything, but of course get a doctor OK first. Just don't give up. You are not alone, there are others like us and it's not in your head.
Author.

Epilogue

I truly believe that until there is a cure for Fibromyalgia, that it helps to share stories of our lives with others who share the same feelings. We have strength in numbers. Plus if we keep talking about it, maybe it will stir up enough noise to get medical science society to make more of an effort to find a cure. We need to be recognized and we need the world to know our pain is real.

Afterward

I am really hoping that the Guaifenesin will work once and for all. I would like to be done with this disease. I am like the rest of you. Tired of being tired. I have had enough **pain** to last me a life time. I now wonder what it would be like to be normal. I question myself. "Have I ever been normal?" "**no**" Thanks for listening.

Conclusions

I hope that the stories that these people have shared will in some way help someone else who is out there alone and afraid. All of us just want you to know that your not alone. We know what you are going through. My sugesetion is that if you get a chance to get on the internet I would do it. You will find so many wonderful friends in the messages boards that will be your friend and help you long your journey.

About the Author

I never really thought of myself as a writer and maybe I am still not. That depends on what the public thinks of my book. I do know that I am very creative and it is my nature to be so. My first love is music. I have my own studio and I have even created my very own CD. It is a collection of my own music that I have written, sang and produced myself. You can find my CD on www.mp3.com under my name, Vance, Dawna. Go to New Artist Search and put my name in if you want to hear some of my music. I have been playing music and singing since I was old enough to walk. My mother can attest to my 2am banging on the piano when I was 3 years old. I once pursued as a career when I was young, but as an adult I gave it up to the real life of living, if you know what I mean. I was voted most likely to suceed in music when I was in school. I would of loved to of been in that world, but I am fully content in doing my own private shows and making my own CD's. Now that I have Fibromyalgia it brought out another creative part in me. I guess that is why I decided to write this book. I thought it would be a great why to express myself and help others at the same time. I really hope you like the book. For me it is a great accomplishment and I am very proud of myself for doing it. Most of all I am proud of making it through all the pain of sitting here day after day. I feel it an inspiration to others. If I can sit here almost in tears and make it, so can you. Good luck to you and thanks again for reading my book.

Notes

My grandmother always said "There is a destoney that makes us brothers, no one goes their way alone. What you put in the life of others comes back into your own." It is my favorite saying.

Jan McDonald has proved her favorites scriptures from the bible in hopes that they might bring a last bit of comfort to those who read my book. Here they are:

As for hope—Psm54:10 "Though the mountains be shaken and the hills be removed, yet my unfailing love for you will not be shaken nor my covenant of peace be removed," says the Lord , who has compassion on you.

Isaiah 40:31 Those who hope in the Lord will renew their strength. They will soar on wings like eagles: they will run and not grow weary, they will walk and not be faint.

Love—1 John 3:1 How great is the love the Father has lavished on us, that we should be called children of God!

John 3:16 For God so loved the world that He gave His only begotten Son, that we should not perish, but have everlasting life.

That verse above is my favorite; it's hope, love, peace and all those rolled into one for me. Thanks for letting me share.

Jan.